SEX—INTERRUPTED

Igniting Intimacy
While Living With Illness
or Disability

SEX—INTERRUPTED

Igniting Intimacy
While Living With Illness
or Disability

By Iris Zink, BSN, MSN, ANP, RN-BC
with Jenny Thorn Palter, BS
and Kirsten Schultz, MS

atmosphere press

TABLE OF CONTENTS

Foreword 3

Introduction 5

What Is Sex—and Why Does It Matter? 8

Iris's Ideas for Maintaining Good Sex and True Intimacy 20

10 Myths Surrounding Sex and Intimacy

1. Sex=Intercourse 32
2. Sex=Orgasm 38
3. General Health Does Not Affect Sexual Health 45
4. Good Sex Just Happens 54
5. Disabled People Are Not Sexual 62
6. There Comes A Time When Sex Is Not Important 69
7. My Health and Physical Changes Have Made Me Unattractive 76
8. I Am Who I Am Sexually Because Of My Parts (Shape, Size, Etc.) 84
9. The Use of Sexual Aids Is Not Sexy 90
10. There Is Nothing More I Can Learn About Sex 104

What Does "Honor Your Partner" Mean? 111

Conclusion 115

The Last Word(s) 117

Appendix A: Personal Lubricants 118

Appendix B: Sexual Orientation 122

Appendix C: Gender Identity 128

Appendix D: Gender and Culture 135

References 137

Recommended Reading 149

Resources 151

Foreword

By Mimi Secor, DNP, FNP-BC, FAANP, FAAN

Individuals with chronic illness or changes to their body are especially vulnerable to loss of sexual expression. Yet the standard educational curricula used to train healthcare providers often neglects the topics of sex and intimacy. Neither is the subject of sexual health regularly addressed in healthcare settings. Understandably, patients may feel uncertain or shy about bringing up the subject of their sexual problems and concerns—especially when chronic health issues give so much else to worry about. All of these factors explain why being able to talk about sexual health with providers, and provider competency in this area, are critical to overall health.

Sex—Interrupted: Igniting Intimacy While Living With Illness or Disability illuminates the importance of addressing patients' sexual health concerns in the safety and privacy of the healthcare provider's office. Written in the direct yet lighthearted manner that reflects how Ms. Zink interacts with her patients and lecture audiences, the book addresses the most common myths about illness and sex. At the same time, it guides and facilitates conversations between providers and patients with a long-term disability or chronic illness. There are also explanations of how providers can give nonjudgmental help to patients, including how to speak in an open, accepting manner while using appropriate terms and easy-to-understand language. Appropriate use of lubricants, sex toys, and physical touch alternatives to intercourse are just a few examples of the topics included.

Yet this book is more than a resource for regaining and maintaining a healthy sex life. By helping us to more confidently discuss the topic of sexual health, the book also enables providers to help patients strengthen, and in many cases heal, intimate relationships that can be so negatively affected by illness or disability. Ultimately, *Sex—Interrupted: Igniting Intimacy While Living With Illness or Disability* encourages providers and patients alike to be more open and confident discussing sex and intimacy, and will help immeasurably to improve the patient-provider relationship.

Introduction

"Not all doctors and nurses are comfortable discussing sexual issues and practices. Most doctors don't routinely ask about your sex life. And patients don't usually begin to discuss their love life with a doctor who hasn't mentioned it. Nobody's talking!" (breastcancer.org, 2019)

In the circle of the holistic self, sexual health has the same importance as the other four components—psychological health, social health, physical health, and spiritual health. Yet sexual health is the least likely component to be discussed in a healthcare setting.

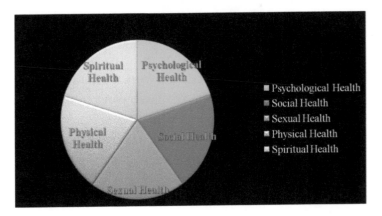

Sexual health is always affected by illness or disability. That is why it's so important for issues of sexual health to be included in any text that offers to help healthcare providers treat and care for people with chronic diseases and disabilities. Yet sexuality, intimacy, and sexual health remain the least likely subjects to be discussed in a healthcare setting, either by the provider or by the patient.

I've had all sorts of people—nuns, nurses, physicians, patients, researchers, and many more—come up to me after one of my lectures and thank me for sharing so much information that was new to them. No, I am not an expert on these topics. And it is not necessary for you to be an expert on sexual matters to have a conversation about sex and intimacy issues, whether with a partner or a healthcare provider. Still, someone must start the conversation!

That "someone" can be you, your healthcare provider, or your partner. But, once the subject is brought up, no matter who is having the discussion, each person needs to know how to listen, and, ideally, the healthcare provider will be able to help with resources and information.

It makes sense to consider this topic from the point of view of those who are affected by some kind of change in their own health or abilities, or by a change that has happened to their partner. To start with, it's natural to feel that your body has truly let you down when you've been diagnosed with a chronic illness or long-term disability. How can you even think about being a sexual person when you're dealing with pain, fatigue, side effects of medications, and the idea of having a disease or an unexpected and unwelcome change to your body for the rest of your life?

Along with learning to cope with the loss of a former healthy life, you may feel anxiety and guilt because you're no longer the same person your partner fell in love with and expects you to be. Changes in each person's role within the relationship, and changes in each partner's perceptions of the other person, cause stress. At the same time, partners face the challenges of what to say, when to touch, and how to help—and they have desires and needs of their own. All of these factors can affect even the most devoted couples.

Gender identity and cultural upbringing are always relevant in any discussion of intimacy and sexuality. We have included a glossary of currently used and no-longer acceptable gender and sexual identity terms and definitions in the Appendices section. Resources concerning cultural mores and beliefs are more difficult to find; we urge anyone interested in learning more to seek out the most recent published research and studies in the journals cited in our reference list, through the American Association of Sexuality Educators, Counselors, and Therapists, and in the other resources listed at the end of the book.

Whether you are a trained healthcare provider, a person living with a chronic illness, or the partner of someone with a disability, our message is simple: Sexual health matters, and help is available. Don't let uncertainty, fear of the unknown, or your current beliefs about the role of intimacy stop you from learning more. What you learn may surprise and delight you!

What is Sex and
Why Does It Matter?

"On one level, sex is just a hormone-driven bodily function designed to perpetuate the species," write the editors in the introduction to the 2015 Harvard Medical School Special Health Report, *Sexuality in Midlife and Beyond*. "But on a higher level, it is an act that embodies the complexity of human physical and emotional responses."

But even among non-humans, sex appears to be regularly practiced—and for a whole range of non-reproductive benefits. Same-sex behavior, including courtship, sexual pair-bonding, and parental activities, has been seen in more than 450 species of animals, notes zoological researcher Bruce Bagemihl in his 2000 book, *Biological Exuberance*. "Male Bonobos kiss ... female Bottlenose Dolphins clasp each other ... male Giraffes engage in 'necking.' ... Sometimes animals gently bite, nibble, or chew on each other's ears (female Hoary Marmots), or wings and chests (Gray-headed Flying Foxes), or rumps (male Dwarf Cavies), or necks (male Savanna Baboons)." Even birds get in the act: "Hammerheads, Acorn Woodpeckers, and Blue-bellied Rollers have ritualized bouts of courtship and mounting activity that may involve groups of individuals and both same-sex and opposite-sex partners."

But it's humans that we want to talk about in this text.

"What sets human sexuality apart from animal and plant sexuality is our capacity—or even drive—to discover how to give and receive pleasure through sexual activity."—ASHA's *Sexual Health Coloring Book*

What actually happens during sex?

From the late 1950s to the mid-1990s, scientists William Masters and Virginia Johnson conducted groundbreaking research that directly observed the physical and physiologic sexual responses of volunteer participants. In doing so, they transformed society's understanding of sexual response and sex therapy. In their invaluable work, they presented the idea of four distinct stages of sexual response, each of which includes anatomic and physiologic changes. The stages are desire, arousal, orgasm, and resolution. (Kinsey Institute, 2018)

According to experts at Harvard Medical School, desire, also known as libido or lust, has three main elements:

- Sexual drive—a hormone-dependent impulse for sexual release (examples: a longing to reproduce, a longing to have sex, erotic thoughts or dreams, an urge to masturbate)
- Sexual wish—the willingness to have sex (to feel more connected to another person, to feel more feminine or masculine, to feel more emotionally alive or physically energetic)
- Sexual motive—the combination of factors that impel a person to want sex (*Sexuality in Midlife and Beyond*, 2015)

Low libido, or lack of desire, is the most challenging form of sexual dysfunction to treat, so all of these elements should be taken into account when examining libido problems.

As for the physiologic changes that occur during the arousal phase, these include:

- Accelerated breathing and heart rate
- Increased muscle tension
- Increased blood flow to the genitals
- Increased body warmth and skin flushing
- Lubrication from the vaginal lining
- Swelling of the labia, clitoris, and upper vagina
- Penile stiffening, along with thickening of the scrotum and drawing in of testicles
- Nipple erections
- Increased sensitivity to stimulation

There are a couple of things to point out about sexual drive, wish, and response. First, people don't have to experience each of the phases in order to enjoy sex. And, women's sexual response patterns may be very different from men's: the four phases may occur in a "non-linear" way for women; and women's responses are more complex than men's. Researcher Rosemary Basson built on the observations of Masters and Johnson by expanding and clarifying women's sexual response during long-term relationships, and by acknowledging that women have a variety of arousal/orgasm responses. Sexuality researchers refer to this as "the Basson Model" (Basson, 2000).

When I give a lecture on sexual health, I always ask the audience this question at the start: "What are the two biggest sex organs in the body?"

It always gets a laugh, but the answer is not a man's penis and a woman's vagina—although that's what most people think.

No, the two biggest sex organs are the skin, the body's largest "organ," and the brain, which decides what turns us on—or doesn't.

If we define sexuality, as do researchers Anita Clayton and Sujatha Ramamurthy, as "the ultimate union of body and mind," then in essence we're talking about skin (body) and brain (mind). But there's much more to it.

"In addition to the biochemical forces at work, your upbringing, experiences, and expectations help shape your sexuality. Your understanding of yourself as a sexual being, your thoughts about what constitutes a satisfying sexual connection, and your relationship with your partner are key factors in your ability to develop and maintain a fulfilling sex life." (*Sexuality in Midlife and Beyond*, Introduction, 2015)

"Sexual health is the ability to embrace and enjoy our sexuality throughout our lives. It is an important part of our physical and emotional health," says The American Sexual Health Association. The ASHA believes that being sexually healthy means:

- Understanding that sexuality is a natural part of life and involves more than sexual behavior.
- Recognizing and respecting the sexual rights we all share.
- Having access to sexual health information, education, and care.
- Making an effort to prevent unintended pregnancies and STDs and seek care and treatment when needed.

- Being able to experience sexual pleasure, satisfaction, and intimacy when desired.
- Being able to communicate about sexual health with others including sexual partners and healthcare providers. (ashasexualhealth.org, 2019)

In 2000, members of the World Health Organization (WHO) and the Pan American Health Organization (PAHO) met to review terminology, identify program options, and develop working definitions of key terms. Representatives from the PAHO and the World Association for Sexual Health (WAS) then met to discuss sexual health issues concerning body integrity, sexual safety, eroticism, gender, sexual orientation, emotional attachment, and reproduction.

The Sexual and Reproductive Health section of the WHO website states that "Sexual health cannot be defined, understood or made operational without a broad consideration of sexuality, which underlies important behaviours and outcomes related to sexual health."

The WHO's current working definition of sexuality is "a central aspect of being human throughout life [that] encompasses sex, gender identities and roles, sexual orientation, eroticism, pleasure, intimacy and reproduction. ... Sexuality is influenced by the interaction of biological, psychological, social, economic, political, cultural, legal, historical, religious and spiritual factors." (WHO.int, 2019)

The definition used by the Come As You Are Co-operative, in its core values and culture statement, states that "Sexuality is part of everyone's experience, regardless of age, gender, race, sexual orientation or identity, disability, ethnicity, religious affiliations, how we move, talk, or think. Celebrating sexuality means embracing the quirkiness in all of us." (ComeAsYouAre.com, 2019)

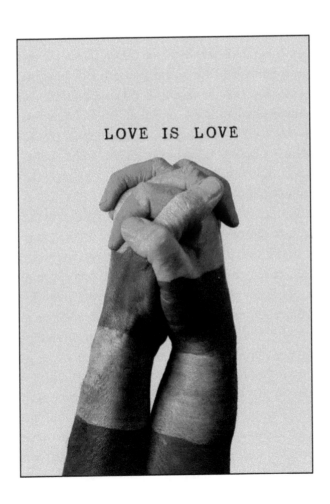

Intimacy

In "Intimacy: The Art of Relationships," published in *Psychology Today* in 2016, researcher Lori H. Gordon writes that, "At the heart of intimacy, then, is empathy, understanding, and compassion; these are the humanizing feelings. ... Sexual problems in a relationship are frequently the by-product of personal and relational conflicts and anxieties. For too many couples, sex has become a substitute for intimacy and a defense against closeness. Most poor sex stems from poor communication, from misunderstandings of what one's mate actually wants—not from unwillingness or inability to give it."

Intimacy brings together the acts of sex (body) and feelings of connectedness and caring (brain). Sometimes it starts with just a touch!

I have a patient, Dolores, who has confided in me that, due to her strong religious beliefs about marriage, she would never seek sex outside her marriage and would not consider leaving her spouse, but he stopped touching her years ago. Dolores has shared with me that this has been so hard on her emotionally and spiritually. She no longer believes she is physically attractive and has often reported feeling undesired or undesirable because of a lack of intimacy in her relationship.

The simplicity of touch creates a bond between two people. "The gentle breath on the back of your neck, a brush of the knee or feather-like kiss on your hand can produce a sexual sensation, depending on who is delivering the touch and to whom," writes Samantha Evans—nurse, sexpert and co-owner of the online sex toy retailer Jo Devine—in her article, "The Lesser Known

Erogenous Zones - And How To Find Them."

Whether the touch is a feather-soft tickle or a suggestive spank depends on what each partner likes.

For many individuals, physical touch is one of the key "languages of love" that they crave. In his 1992 book *The Five Love Languages: How to Express Heartfelt Commitment to Your Mate*, author Gary Chapman writes, "People experience love most strongly through one of five love languages—quality time, words of encouragement, gifts, acts of service, and physical touch."

Touch as part of intimacy can be thrilling or exploratory, suggestive or demanding. Touch:

- Provides a connection
- Conveys affirmation
- Reassures
- Decreases stress
- Improves self-esteem

What feels good?

OK, now another quiz question. If I ask you to name the erogenous zones of the human body, what would you include in your list? Common answers are mouth, breasts, and genitals. Fair enough. But think about this: Those suggestions neglect all the other parts of the body that can produce a sexual response! What about feet, ears, and the sides and back of the neck, or the inside of the arm? And what about what happens when you look deeply into someone's eyes?

The WebMD article "7 Awesome Erogenous Zones" adds a few more: the inner wrist, the scalp, behind the knee, and the buttocks.

In "The Lesser Known Erogenous Zones—And How To Find Them," Samantha Evans writes, "Understanding erogenous zones is ... important to people who experience decreased sexual sensation as a result of illness, disease, disability, injury or following surgery to ensure that they can still enjoy sexual pleasure and function. This also applies to people undergoing gender reassignment surgery or breast augmentation."

An excellent way to find out what each partner enjoys is trying what Ms. Evans calls "body mapping"—"a simple self-exploration technique in which people who experience decreased sexual sensation (as a result of conditions such as multiple sclerosis) can enjoy sexual pleasure." This technique uses gentle touch on all parts of the body to help each partner identify areas of sensual pleasure, as well as any areas of discomfort.

The authors of *Sexuality in Midlife and Beyond* stress that pleasure can be experienced without genital-to-genital contact: "Pleasurable activities—from intimacies such as kissing and caressing to more intense types of physical contact designed to produce orgasm—can complement intercourse or stand alone as a means for gratification." They explain that, whether partners focus on the mouth, the breasts, the anal area, the hands, feet, or other sensitive spots on each other's skin, it's really all about giving and receiving pleasure. Furthermore, sexual activity can be enjoyed solo, via masturbation, the use of sexually stimulating materials, and personal fantasies. (Harvard Health, 2015)

Is sex good for us?

From WebMD to CNN.com, from the *Journal of the American Medical Association* to the International Society of Sexual Medicine, the answer seems to be a resounding "YES!"

Going back in time a bit, we can reference the *TIME* magazine Special Issue of January 19, 2004, titled "How Your Love Life Keeps You Healthy." Among the articles in the section, which ranged from mating and the science of lust, to what exactly happens in the brain, is a two-page piece called "Sexual Healing." In it, we learn that sexual activity benefits the body in areas as diverse as heart disease, weight, pain, depression, anxiety, immunity, cancer, and longevity.

WebMD, in the 2013 article, "10 Surprising Health Benefits of Sex," lists these results:

1. Helps keep your immune system humming
2. Boosts your libido
3. Improves women's bladder control
4. Lowers your blood pressure
5. Counts as exercise
6. Lowers heart attack risk
7. Lessens pain
8. May make prostate cancer less likely
9. Improves sleep
10. Eases stress

The article concludes by saying, "Sex and intimacy can boost your self-esteem and happiness, too ... It's not only a prescription for a healthy life, but a happy one."

A National Social Life, Health and Aging Project study

of several thousand older women and men revealed benefits to women's cardiovascular health from a rewarding sexual relationship—at the same time noting that women are especially vulnerable to cardiovascular problems from poor relationship quality or marital loss. (Liu et al, 2016)

I know some people have concerns about engaging in sexual activities after having a heart event. But as a healthcare provider, I believe it's safe to say that, as long as you can climb a flight of stairs without a problem, you should be fine to engage in sex. Consider sex as the most enjoyable workout ever devised.

And then, sex is—or should be—fun! Sure, gardening, traveling, and playing cards are fun, too, but don't usually cause your heart to start racing!

Besides being good for physical health, sexual satisfaction is important for psychological health. In a large study of U.S. adults' ratings of the importance of sexual health and satisfaction with sex life, sexual health was found to be a highly important aspect of quality of life for many participants, including those in poor health. (Flynn et al, 2016)

At the same time, knowledge of one's sexuality and an understanding of how to be sexually healthy can have a positive impact early on. "Positive sexually related experiences in romantic relationships during adolescence may complement physical, mental/emotional, and social health," was the conclusion of a 10-year longitudinal cohort study of sexual relationships and sexual behavior among adolescent women.

The study also noted that healthcare providers, by discussing specific aspects of healthy sexual development with their adolescent patients, could at the same time address other common adolescent health issues. (Hensel, Nance, and Fortenberry, 2016)

Iris's Ideas for Maintaining Good Sex and True Intimacy

When intimacy and sexual expression have been adversely affected by illness or loss, don't despair. By making yourself open to asking questions and sharing what you learn with your partner or, if you're a healthcare provider, with your patients, a couple's closeness and sexual energy can be regained, and even improved. We'll explore all of these in other ways throughout this book, but here are the ideas I think are most important.

1. Don't be afraid to bring up the subject of sex and intimacy. Talking about sexual issues isn't the easiest thing in the world, and if you feel like you can't talk to your partner, maybe you'll find it easier to ask questions and ask for help in the privacy of the exam room. Your healthcare provider may be able to help you. If not, ask for a referral to someone who can help.

Nisha McKenzie, PA-C, CSC, IF, founder and director of the Center for Women's Sexual Health in Grand Rapids, MI, and Justine Braford, LMSW, CST, founder of Grand Rapids Specialty Therapy, find that the most common sexual health concerns among their female patients are:

- Lack of desire/desire discrepancy between partners
- Difficulty with arousal
  - Lack of wetness
  - Slow to get in the mood
  - Difficulty getting/maintaining erections

- o Taking a long time to ejaculate/reach orgasm
- Genito-pelvic pain and penetration disorders
  - o Dyspareunia (painful intercourse) due to atrophy
  - o Vaginismus (overtight vaginal muscle)
  - o Overactive pelvic floor (can cause muscle spasm)
  - o Vestibulodynia (pain in the vulva)
- Primary versus secondary anorgasmia (never experiencing orgasm under any circumstances vs. experiencing orgasm but having concerns with frequency or circumstances of occurrence)
- Lack of pleasure from sex

2. Know where to go for help. Many different kinds of healthcare providers are trained to address sexual rehabilitation and other sexual health-related issues. These providers are usually found at medical facilities with a broad range of healthcare services.

- Nurses are critical in assisting with the overall medical management of a disability. Nurses also help with the execution of many of the suggestions given by the different therapists, physicians, or other clinicians.
- Sexual Health Clinicians are nurses specialized in the area of sexual health. They are experts in educating clients and their partners on the complex changes to sexual function as a result of chronic illness or disability, and they are qualified to make specific suggestions to

enhance sexual functioning and/or fertility.

- Sexual Medicine Physicians or Physiatrists can assist with maximizing sexual physiology and reducing the medical issues that often interfere with sexual interest and activities; other physicians (urologist, gynecologist, neurologist, etc.) may also have valuable expertise.

- Occupational Therapists help enable clients to manage and perform their daily activities. OTs can address issues around sexuality. OTs can also adapt sexual devices to meet the abilities of clients (e.g., adding switches, making "hands free" options, etc.).

- Physical therapists (also called Physiotherapists) address clients' physical function and can help with range of motion, pelvic muscle strength, and other movement-related issues.

- Social Workers can play a large role in educating and counseling partners and families around sexual and fertility issues.

- Psychologists explore in depth with clients the many different emotional components of sexuality such as self-esteem, assertiveness, and positive self-talk, and can also address trauma around sexuality.

- Recreational Therapists work with clients to explore meaningful recreation and leisure choices. Friendship development through involvement in recreation activities of mutual interest is often key to meeting potential partners. The National Council for Therapeutic Recreation Certification also notes that Therapeutic Recreation helps individuals with illnesses or disabling conditions seeking to recover their psychological and physical health and well-being.

- Peer Counselors, such as persons with disabilities themselves, are critical sources of information and support, and are the experts on what their bodies experience. (from "PleasureABLE"—a sexual device manual for persons with disabilities, 2009, and nctrc.org/about-ncrtc/, 2020).

3. Stay informed about your, and your partner's, sexual health history. Sally Pelon, PhD, and Lihua Huang, PhD, professors in the School of Social Work at Grand Valley State University in Grand Rapids, Michigan, believe that healthcare providers should begin with "complete and compassionate history-taking." They compiled these questions as a guide for healthcare providers with new patients, but for our own health and well-being, each of us should also know our own history. It's also a good idea to have a conversation about sexual health history with a new sexual partner.

- Are you currently sexually active?
- Are you currently sexually active with more than one partner?
- What kinds of protection do you and your partner(s) use during sexual activity?
- How has your illness or disease affected your sexual activity?

- How have your medications affected your sexual activity?
- Have you ever had a sexually transmitted disease, or knowingly been exposed to a sexually transmitted disease?
- Have you ever had, or do you now have any discharge, rash, or sores in your genital area?
- Are there any sexual issues you would like to talk about?

They also offer these recommendations to healthcare providers:

- Check your assumptions, such as assumed heterosexuality, assumed monogamy, celibacy in single women, and the importance of sexuality.
- Walk alongside the individual or couple—not behind or in front.
- Don't underestimate the importance of education, including terminology, anatomy, and specific facts about sex.
- Conduct a physical exam.
- Slowly complete a psychosocial history, over several meetings.
- Include grief work over what's been lost.
- Encourage individuals to draw upon resiliencies that already exist from a lifetime of coping.

By including sexual health questions in each patient visit, healthcare providers will be able to respond quickly to questions and to help with existing or new problems. An individual's attachment history, sexual history, relationship history, and trauma history can be uncovered over time once the person feels safe and secure.

4. Practice safe sex. And on the subject of sexual health history, perhaps nothing is so imperative for sexually active adults as an understanding of safe sex. It's well worth remembering that, when a partner's HIV, Hepatitis C, and STI (sexually transmitted infection) status is unknown, there is a risk of STI transmission. The best way to avoid getting an STI is to avoid sexual contact altogether. This advice is not always realistic, of course. The risk of infection transmission can be lessened by practicing smart sex and engaging in the least risky behavior until the partner's STI status is known. That's why it's so important to prepare for sexual contact ahead of time. This list explains the relative safety of common sexual activities:

- *Very Safe.* Mutual masturbation is the safest form of sexual contact, allowing for sexual pleasure without the risk of STI transmission. Participants should take care to prevent transmission of blood or bodily fluids directly into or near the vaginal opening. Making sure hands and fingernails are clean will lower the risk of bacteria being introduced into the vagina or anus during finger penetration.
- *Mostly Safe.* Oral sex is the next least risky behavior for reducing transmission of an STI— as long as there are no cuts or sores on the mouth or genitals. Each participant will want

to visually inspect all partners before starting oral sex. It's also recommended that participants avoid brushing teeth or flossing immediately before oral sex; this is because any abrasions of the mouth's mucosa can allow infection to pass to a partner. It's especially important that anyone with periodontal disease avoids participating in oral sex, due to the imbalance of bacterial flora and increased risk of infection. Note: Barrier devices such as dental dams and condoms can further reduce risk of STI transmission.

- *Safe If Used with a Barrier Method.* If engaging in vaginal penetrative sex with a partner whose STI status is unknown, use of a barrier method, such as male or female condom, is best practice. If a condom is not available, use of a lubricant is recommended to reduce the number of microtears that occur during intercourse, which can then become portals of transmission for bacteria and viruses. There are many types of lubricants available; however, oil-based lubes are not recommended for use with barrier methods.

- *Risky.* Anal sex is the riskiest behavior in which to participate if one is unaware of a partner's STI status, because the thin layers of anal mucosa tear easily, which then allow viruses and bacteria to enter the body. Lubricants and condoms can lessen the risk of STI transmission. Pre-exposure prophylaxis (PrEP)—which is daily oral medication for those at high risk for HIV—will lower the chances of HIV transmission for those who engage in anal sex. Together, PrEP and condoms further reduce STI transmission rate. Additional information and resources can be found on the CDC's website in the "Act Against AIDS" section, featuring a campaign called "Start Talking. Stop HIV."

5. Talk to your partner. Intuitively, we know that there's a need for intimacy among partners. Yet it can be hard to know what to say to a partner, and when to say it; it can also be hard to be a good listener, and it can be hard, sometimes, to know how to receive what we hear.

Talk with your clothes on first! Start with the word "I":

- I've noticed ...
- I like it when we ...
- I like it when you touch me ...
- I would really like to try _____
- I heard about a study where people _____

This is also a time to be honest—with yourself and with your partner.

- Get to know the sexual parts of your own body and your partner's body; know what arouses each of you.
- Talk to your partner about what makes you aroused. (If you're interested in steamy sex talk, you have to practice!)
- Help your partner understand what feels good to you. And if something doesn't feel good to you, tell your partner that, too.

- Most of all, make your time together a priority.

Each of us is an individual, and each individual has a personal and particular relationship to the world at large. When you talk about what's bothering you, you may find that your concerns are the same as other people who are in intimate relationships:

- Your physical appearance and how you appear to your partner and to others
- Your feelings about sex and how your partner feels about sex
- Your thoughts about the kind of sex life you have
- The frequency of sex in your relationship, and whether it's right for your partner

6. Stay informed. Recommended reading, websites, organizations, and sexual health experts are listed after the Resources section at the end of this book. Search for "sexual health and ..." rather than "sex and ..." on the internet. Self-care and stress management are equally important! In addition, understanding one's own body (self-touch) can enhance one's sex life. Partners should take the opportunity to talk about sex during the office visit, and to ask for evidence-based suggestions that they can try at home. Nobody wants to be seen as dumb about sex, so all parties should try to stay respectful when providing and receiving information: "As perhaps you already know ..." or "My spouse wants to try ..." or "I read about ... Do you know anything about that?" A healthcare provider who addresses anxieties first has a chance to normalize the discussions; for example: "Many people experience this ...”

7. Acknowledge grief and loss. Many of us are familiar with Dr. Elizabeth Kübler-Ross's stages of grief: denial, anger, bargaining, depression, and acceptance. When we experience a loss or change in health, whether it happens to us or to our partner, it is necessary to allow for these feelings in order to recover and rebuild our life and our intimate relationship.

People grieve losses in different ways, but it's always advisable to use our survival skills, and to practice gratitude for family and relationships. Instead of pulling away in loss, we should try to find appreciation for those who stood by us in our time of need and who continue to stand by us in life—not just in times of illness.

Dr. Allen Klein, author of *Learning to Laugh When You Feel Like Crying: Embracing Life After Loss*, suggests five steps for moving on after grieving:

1. Losing
2. Learning
3. Letting go
4. Living
5. Laughing

8. Be sensitive to sexual orientation and gender identity. People deserve to be able to talk candidly with their healthcare providers without fear of judgement or misunderstanding or rejection. That kind of respect must start at the first meeting and must continue throughout the course of the patient-provider relationship. It's totally acceptable to ask for the preferred personal pronouns if unsure. Appendices B, C, and D contain up-to-date definitions as well as acceptable and non-acceptable terms.

Putting it all together

As with all things, communication is key to understanding what each person wants and needs in a sexual relationship. In real estate, it's all about "location, location, location." Well, in sex, it's all about "communication, communication, communication!" Here are some ideas for anyone who isn't sure how to get the conversation going:

- Start a journal to help you put your feelings into words that you can share.
- At a place and time you won't be interrupted, talk to your partner about your shared sex life. Start the conversation with a neutral topic—something you read or saw on TV about intimacy and sex.
- Reassure your partner that you're asking about their feelings because you really want to know.
- Talk, pause, and ask for feedback—use eye contact and touch to reinforce what you say.
- Consider getting help from a licensed sex therapist.
- And remember: Whether or not intimacy leads to intercourse or orgasm, the important thing is that you are paying attention to each other and reinforcing your "togetherness."

This acronym sums up what I think are important for each of us as we pursue a satisfying sex life:

S – **S**elf-confidence—**S**ense of **S**elf

H – A sense of **H**umor

E – **E**nthusiasm—drive and desire

E – **E**ducation

T – **T**ools—and a good support network

S – **S**pirit—and patience!

In the words of philosopher and author Bertrand Russell, "Those who have never known the deep intimacy and the intense companionship of happy mutual love have missed the best thing that life has to give." (1929)

In the next section, we'll examine and explore 10 myths about sex. You may recognize some of these as myths, but I hope you'll learn some things that will surprise and enlighten you, too.

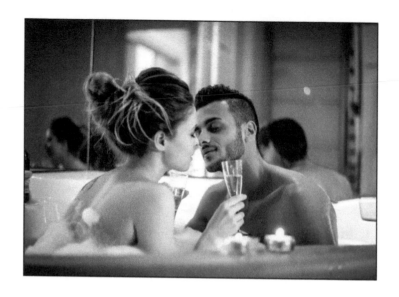

Myth #1: Sex = Intercourse

"Vaginal intercourse is often given a lofty position as the ultimate sexual event, but clearly the story doesn't begin or end there."—Harvard Health Publications, 2015

The definition of sex for individuals changes over time due to health issues or changes in desires. Yet it's important to realize that losing the ability to maintain an erection or to tolerate penetration does not make us any less sexual. Sexual expression evolves out of necessity—and desire. If there can be said to be a goal for sex, it would have to be true intimacy.

For example, in a study that examined attitudes and feelings of men who had undergone prostatectomy, the researchers found that many of the men were very worried about no longer being able to satisfy their partners—yet their wives and girlfriends didn't see it that way at all. One woman explained that it was "incredibly important" for her partner to understand that "there are plenty of ways to please her that she's happy to show him and that they can learn together. The most important thing for her is that they stay physically connected." (Alterowitz and Alterowitz, 2018)

This quote is from an article on resuming a healthy sex life after cancer, but it applies just as well to any couple dealing with a life-changing illness or disease: "The couples who rehabilitate intimacy together are the couples with a good shot at having great sex. Perhaps even more importantly, they're also the ones who more often describe the results as truly great sex." (Cavanaugh, 2015)

Marlene, a young woman in her early 30s, came to see me for lupus and Sjögren's syndrome. She was steroid-dependent due to the severity of her lupus, and she had previously shared with me that her husband, Andrew, had prostate problems. She told me she was trying to keep life as normal as possible, but they hadn't had any kind of sex for two years.

She said that recently they decided to take a cruise, and, unbeknownst to her, Andrew had brought along some Viagra, and one night he came out of the bathroom with a huge erection, expecting her to be ready, willing, and able to enjoy a night of passion—but he hadn't talked to her about it at all.

"I was petrified with worry and fear that penetration would really hurt after so long," Marlene told me, "and my husband was mortified when he understood how I felt."

It certainly wasn't the steamy lovemaking scene he had envisioned.

Lesson learned: Being able to talk about sex and what each partner is feeling, and expecting, ahead of time, gives each person the chance to be prepared, and will likely lead to a very different (and much more satisfying) encounter.

Women often need more than a casual "Let's do this!" to become sexually aroused. That means, the more time a woman has to think about sex, the more likely it is that she's going to want to have sex, and the more fun it will be for both partners. Here are a few pretty good ideas for getting in the mood:

- When you're not together, use texting and emails to send each other little stories to keep things exciting.
- Foreplay helps both mentally and physically—especially for women. Try spending 30 minutes touching each other without engaging in intercourse or trying for an orgasm; you may find that the anticipation really heats things up for both of you.
- It may be necessary for a woman to use a vaginal moisturizer or lubricant during intercourse if she has Sjögren's syndrome (which causes dryness in the moisture-producing glands) or if she's post-menopausal (which causes lower estrogen levels and decreased blood supply to the vagina, leading to thinner, dryer vaginal tissue).
  - Products that moisturize and lubricate are Replens® long-lasting vaginal inserts, Lubrin® vaginal lubricating inserts, and Aloe Cadabra® liquid.

- o Products that offer short-term lubrication include Just Like Me® gel from Pure Romance (request their catalog), K-Y® jelly or beads, and Astroglide®.
- o Prescription products include Vagifem® inserts and estrogen cream or rings.
- Share some of the sex advice in *Cosmopolitan* magazine, grab a copy of the 2011 erotic romance bestseller, *50 Shades of Grey* by E.L. James, or rent the film, or pick a different sexy movie. Or you might want to try making up your own sexy stories.
- Come up with a cue that alerts your partner when you're in the mood for sex. Think of it as a mating call! Just remember—it's an opportunity for intimacy.
- If illness, medication side effects, fatigue, or other concerns are preventing you from feeling sexual, remember that intimacy takes many forms—from listening to music together, holding hands at the movies, going for a walk in the park, getting a couples massage, sharing a shower or bubble bath, or even just "spooning" in bed with no clothes on. Think back to the days when you were first dating and recreate your favorite experiences together.
- If you're interested in steamy sex talk, practice!
- Being distracted during intimacy is an example of not being in the moment. In meditation, you learn to redirect your brain to focus on your

senses. It's the same with intimacy—your partner's scent, the feeling of touching each other's skin, the heat of a body near yours, and the tastes and sight of your partner all work together to produce intimacy. When you're not fully involved in enjoying the close bond of intimacy with your partner, orgasm will be a difficult or even unachievable goal.

- Date! Make it a priority!
- Try to get in some kind of physical exercise each day—it really does makes you feel better.

"Sex isn't just penis in vagina; it's all kinds of other activities, too!" say the experts at breastcancer.org. The online site SmartSexResource offers a good list of alternatives to intercourse:

- Kissing
- Hand jobs/fingering
- Self-pleasure—masturbation and mutual masturbation
- Sexual rubbing without penetration (also called dry humping or "frottage")
- Nipple play
- Sex toy play
- Tantric sex—a practice that involves slower touch, massage or meditation, with a focus on breath, connection, and sensations
- Phone sex/sexting
- Online sex

Oral sex isn't included but is also an alternative.

The added bonus of experimenting with alternatives

to intercourse is an expansion of each person's understanding of what the other person likes.

"Outercourse"—as it's sometimes called—also provides safe sex when there's a lack of knowledge of a partner's STID (sexually transmitted infectious disease) status.

Adopting a "conscious, intentional approach by engaging in regular sexual stimulation in order to enjoy sexual expression" was the finding of a study of how couples learn to recover their sex lives following prostatectomy. (Wittmann et al, 2015)

Ruth and Glenn were in my exam room one morning. I know Glenn smokes, so whenever there's a smoking person in the room I ask about impotence, because we know that smoking can contribute to impotence.

I asked the couple, "How's your sex life?"

Glenn looked down and then at Ruth, and said to me, "Well, ask my wife."

She said to me, "No, ask him."

I looked again at Glenn and he said, "Well, you know, since my prostate cancer nothing much works down there."

I looked over at Ruth and said, "His tongue broke when he had prostate surgery."

They both started laughing, and she slapped his leg and said, "See, I told we could still have sex, I told you!"

Lesson learned: Many times, we automatically think "intercourse is sex, end of story." But there are many different kinds of sex.

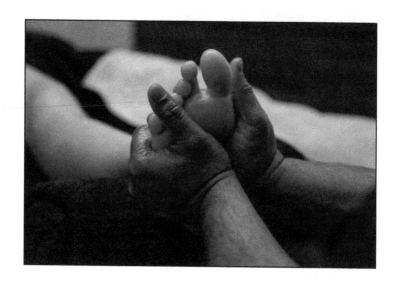

Myth #2: Sex = Orgasm

"Orgasms are like icing on cake. Cake is great by itself, and sometimes there isn't time, or there are too many distractions, for an orgasm to happen—but 'cake sex' is important for bonding. The 'orgasm icing' just makes it better."—Iris Zink, 2019

The "goal" of sex is not orgasm any more than the goal of sex is intercourse. The truth is, some people no longer have the ability to achieve orgasm due to health conditions and/or medication side effects. Even in the context of perfect health, orgasm is not possible for everyone. Think of the ability to achieve orgasm as a bell curve: On the end of the curve are those who can have lots of orgasms, and on the other end of the curve are those who have never experienced an orgasm.

In a letter to his wife's gynecologist, a husband wrote, "My wife had a total hysterectomy about three years ago, and since her surgery she has not been able to achieve orgasm.... This has been devastating to my ego and has caused my own erectile dysfunction problems."

This man believed that his sole reason for having sex with his wife was to make her orgasm—that it was the one thing he did for her that made him feel good about himself, and also to make her feel really loved.

"I still love my wife very much and always will, but the spark and excitement is gone," he concluded.

The man's concern and grief are genuine, but the gynecologist asked him to reconsider his reaction, and pointed out the overarching importance of intimacy: "I applaud your desire to make sure that your wife is satisfied. I am concerned, however, that your self-esteem appears to be tied to the sexual response of your wife. Every person is responsible for his or her own sexual experience. You can't wrap an orgasm up in a little blue box and hand it to her. You may use techniques that assist her along the way, but you can't control it or will it to happen. And if she feels pressured to perform sexually, it will become even harder for her to experience pleasure or orgasm again."

The gynecologist went on to suggest that the man shift his focus to helping his wife have the best sexual experience that she can, rather than expecting her to have any particular response.

"Chances are, with relaxation, patience, experimentation, and exploration, her ability to achieve orgasm will return," the doctor said. "Remember, sex is so much more than orgasm. Intimacy alone is very important in a marriage." (Hutcherson, 2011)

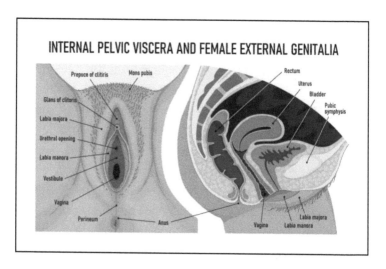

INTERNAL PELVIC VISCERA AND FEMALE EXTERNAL GENITALIA

Tina is a 45-year-old woman who came to me after being told by her primary care doctor that she had systemic lupus. We rechecked her labs and she did have an autoimmune disease, but it was Sjögren's syndrome, not lupus. I educated Tina on the signs and symptoms of Sjögren's and explained that the disease affects the moisture-producing glands of the body, so she was going to have to take extra good care of her teeth (see a dentist every 3-4 months); her eyes (see an ophthalmologist at least twice a year, and use wetting drops daily); and her vagina (use plenty of the right kind of lubrication).

When I asked her if she had noticed any vaginal dryness, she changed the subject. So, I circled back and asked point-blank, "Are you having any issues with intercourse due to vaginal dryness?"

Tina said she had stopped having intercourse with her

husband about two years ago due to, in her words, "just not being able to feel anything down there anymore."

"But you used to be able to orgasm and had previously enjoyed sex?" I asked.

She said, "Yes, early on, but the last few years sex and intimacy has become more of a chore due to fatigue and my lack of pleasure with intercourse."

I then talked to her about neuropathy (lack of sensation to the clitoris and vaginal area due to decreased blood flow or nerve damage), what it was, and how common the symptoms were in all autoimmune diseases, including lupus, rheumatoid arthritis, and especially Sjögren's syndrome. I educated her that sex could still be very enjoyable, but she would need a lot more stimulation.

"Do you miss the intimacy? What about your husband?" I asked.

"Ted stopped even initiating sex when my joint pain and fatigue started; he said he didn't want to make me feel any more pain than I was already experiencing," she told me.

"That was completely normal," I said, "but it doesn't have to continue that way."

We discussed how she could talk to Ted and things that they could try. I gave her a Pure Romance catalog that I had, as well as a sex therapist referral card, and I encouraged her to bring up the subject of intimacy with her husband.

"But before trying any sexual stimulation, you're going to need to use lots of lubrication and start regular Kegel exercises to help with blood flow," I explained. "With Sjögren's the vaginal tissue can get really dry and brittle, and any tiny tears in the mucosa can lead to pain and infection. That's why lubrication is a must with any sexual activity and has to be reapplied often."

Tina returned in six weeks for her checkup. I asked her how things were going, and she reported that she had spoken to her husband and that they were taking things slowly.

"I'm really worried that if we have intercourse that I won't be able to have an orgasm and my husband will feel let down," she admitted.

We talked again about lubrication and about how blood flow can come from stimulation, and that she would need as much blood flow as possible in order to experience an orgasm.

I normalized the situation by saying, "What you're experiencing is not just due to your Sjögren's—lots of men and women struggle with orgasm issues after age 40. Our bodies change and so must how we stimulate them. You'll need a lot of stimulation to have an orgasm. That stimulation could come from your husband's mouth, or hands. Or, a vibrator. Have you ever used a vibrator or practiced self-stimulation?"

She shook her head several times at that. "I grew up as a Jehovah's Witness and I was preached to over and over about the sins of masturbation," she said. It was yet another hurdle.

"Have you looked at the Pure Romance Catalogue or called the sexual therapist?"

She said she felt uncomfortable doing that. She paused, and then she said, "Maybe this isn't really that important."

I used the silent technique.

She looked at me and asked me, "What do you think?"

I used my kitchen example. "I don't cook without OXO brand tools, which help to make food prep easier," I said. "Instead of chopping vegetables by hand, you sometimes use the food processor, right? Well, sometimes you need a tool in the bedroom."

That made her smile.

On Tina's next visit, her husband Ted came with her. She introduced him to me, and he shook my hand and said, "I wanted to meet the woman who gave me back my wife."

Ted said that all he wanted was for Tina to feel better. He said her fatigue and joint pain were improved and that having her back to her old self made him feel better too.

I asked about their sex life.

"We're taking things slowly, but we hug, kiss, and hold hands a lot more," Ted told me.

And then he said, "I'm not afraid to touch her anymore."

I suggested that they follow up with me as needed and to let me know if there was any other support I could give.

Lesson learned: Sometimes it can take a few discussions to really understand what's going on with a patient, and sometimes a few more to see that change is taking place.

Although orgasm does not have to be the goal, nevertheless many people do desire to reach, and help their partner reach, this kind of climax during their lovemaking.

Current research has revealed that women are able to experience orgasms from a variety of "triggering zones" including the external clitoral glans, the region around the G-spot that corresponds to the internal clitoral bulbs, the cervix, and non-genital areas such as the nipples. Partners will discover that stimulating these areas, along with sensory inputs, movements, body positions, autonomic (involuntary) arousal, and partner- and contextual-related cues, will help to bring pleasure and orgasm during masturbation and intercourse. (Pfaus et al, 2016)

In other encouraging research news, orgasm was found to inhibit pain in a 2017 study of 10 women. While the women manually reached a climax alone and with a partner's help, an MRI scanner was used to observe their brains. The scans showed that the part of the brain that helps control serotonin—the chemical that acts to lessen pain sensations—became activated during orgasm. Extra activity also was seen in the area of the brain stem that's believed to affect our ability to control pain deliberately.

"Together, this activity—at least in part—seems to account for the pain-attenuating effect of the female orgasm," says Nan Wise, one of the Rutgers University study's investigators.

It's not necessary to bring a partner to orgasm in order to give pleasure, though. Helping around the house, a foot massage at the end of a long day, spooning while falling asleep—these and similar small acts can be just as appreciated as an orgasm—maybe even more. (Hutcherson, 2011)

Chocolate, meditation, singing, group prayer, and exercise also increase serotonin, as do antidepressants, so if you're having a down day, try an orgasm—it's calorie-free and feels better. Burn calories—have more sex!

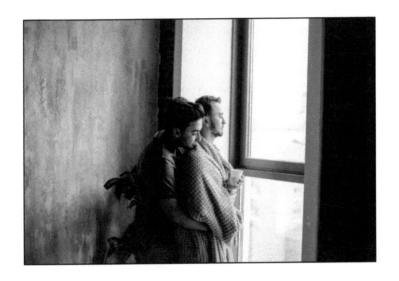

Myth #3: General Health Does Not Affect Sexual Health

"We can continue to be limited by a fantasy view of what bodies are like and what sex is, one that marginalises most of us at some point, or we can grow up and start to accept each other and ourselves."—Aly Fixter, 2019

According to the Partnership to Fight Chronic Disease, nearly 60% of all Americans have at least one chronic condition, and many have two or more. Nearly one in two working-age adults (45-64) have more than one chronic condition, and nearly one in five 18- to 44-year-olds have more than one chronic condition.

Medical disorders that impair blood supply or cause innervation of genital tissue are associated with lack of sexual interest, arousal and orgasmic disorders, as well as general discomfort with sex. (Pelon and Huang, 2019)

Many health conditions can affect sexual health, but even this long list is not exhaustive.

Physical, Emotional, and Mental Conditions That Affect Sexual Health

- Arthritis
- Asthma/pulmonary disease
- Blindness
- Benign prostatic hyperplasia (BPH) surgery
- Cancer, especially of the breast, the reproductive organs, and the prostate
- Cardiovascular disease (CVD)/post-myocardial infarction (MI) or cerebrovascular accident (CVA)
- Chronic obstructive pulmonary disease (COPD/emphysema)
- Chronic pain
- Cognitive impairment and dementia
- Cutaneous lupus erythematosus (CLE)
- Deafness
- Dementia
- Depression
- Dermatomyositis (DM)
- Diabetes
- Dyspareunia
- Erectile dysfunction (ED)
- Fibromyalgia syndrome (FMS)
- HIV/AIDS
- Hypertension (HTN)
- Incontinence

- Inflammatory bowel diseases (Crohn's disease, ulcerative colitis)
- Interstitial cystitis
- Multiple sclerosis (MS)
- Osteoarthritis
- Parkinson's disease
- Psoriasis/eczema/neurofibromatosis
- Rheumatoid arthritis (RA)
- Sjögren's syndrome
- Sleep apnea
- Spinal cord injury
- Stroke
- Systemic lupus erythematosus (SLE)
- Vulvodynia

Being diagnosed with any illness or condition that affects a person's health changes the dynamic of the relationship and can put stress on every aspect of the relationship, from physical to emotional. And it's not only people in relationships who are affected.

For example, research published in the journal *Cancer* revealed that adolescents derive a great deal of their self-esteem from their own sexual identity. When faced with cancer during this time in their lives, adolescents can develop a negative sexual identity.

"Obstacles in accessing sexual-health knowledge, difficulties in interpersonal relationships, and body image concerns may be hurdles that adolescents and young adults with cancer confront in pursuit of sexual health, which may, in turn, hamper the development of a positive self-esteem." (Evan et al, 2006).

Jasmine was one of the first patients I met as a rheumatology Nurse Practitioner. She was being seen in our clinic for fibromyalgia and chronic pain. When I met Jasmine, I loved her instantly. She had a remarkably high-stress job, had had a rough childhood, and was clearly a no-nonsense woman. After hearing her story, it wasn't hard to understand why she had become distrustful of the medical community.

She was taking morphine, and when I asked why she had been prescribed morphine, she replied, "My crotch has nerve damage from a bad hysterectomy. The pain is like a hot knife being stabbed into my labia." She added that there were many nights the pain kept her from sleeping.

She told me that she had gone back to her Ob/Gyn and was told that the pain was due to swelling and should resolve. Instead, the nerve and groin pain intensified. She sought a second opinion, but still got no answers. She was finally referred to a pain specialist who ordered an EMG of her pelvic floor, and the imaging revealed nerve damage from her hysterectomy.

The specialist thought that if the nerve could be isolated and blocked with an epidural or nerve block procedure, maybe Jasmine would have an end to the pain. Unfortunately, the problem was more complicated than expected: The damaged nerve was the same one that innervates (supplies activity to) her bladder. So, blocking this nerve would result in loss of bladder control. That avenue was closed. Jasmine started taking morphine for the pain, and since she also had pain due to fibromyalgia she came to our rheumatology clinic for ongoing pain management.

I asked more about the pain and then curiosity got the best of me. I said, "Can you have sex?"

"No," she said, "it's way too painful," and she started to cry. She talked about how hard this whole thing had been on her relationship with her husband and how she missed the intimacy and felt like she had lost her connection with him. She was worried that he would divorce her or seek intimacy elsewhere.

I said: "It's time to problem-solve."

We decided to try lidocaine jelly; she would apply it liberally to her vaginal area and have her husband wear a condom so he would not become numb as well. She said she understood that she would be numb, but she still wanted to enjoy the closeness with her husband. She was excited to give it a try.

Two weeks later I saw her at a return visit. This woman who had such a hard, stoic exterior grabbed me and hugged me, and her eyes welled up with tears. "We had sex and it was great!" she said. "It didn't hurt near as much as I thought it would."

Jasmine continues to take pain medication and gabapentin for the chronic nerve pain, but over the years that I've been seeing her she says she's been able to remain intimate with her husband and that they've found new creative ways to experience closeness.

One aspect of chronic illness that we should always be aware of is that people who have been diagnosed with a chronic illness will feel the loss of their previous health. Because of this, they find themselves facing stages of grief.

"The five stages—denial, anger, bargaining, depression and acceptance—are a part of the framework that makes up our learning to live with [loss]," writes David Kessler, co-author with Dr. Kübler-Ross of *On Grief and Grieving: Finding the Meaning of Grief Through the Five Stages of Loss* (2014).

"These stages are tools to help us frame and identify what we may be feeling. But they are not stops on some linear timeline in grief. Not everyone goes through all of them or in a prescribed order."

Not just the loss but the recovery can include feelings of grief, according to a study of couples' sexual recovery after surgery for prostate cancer. "Grief was a salient feature of the recovery process," noted the researchers of the study. "Anticipatory grief was reported prior to surgery, while grief related to actual losses was reported after surgery." (Wittmann et al, 2015)

Maria, age 35, was experiencing urinary incontinence. "I'm embarrassed to have intercourse or be intimate with my husband because I lose control of my urine," she told me at her visit.

She added that the incontinence during physical activity was also making her feel apprehensive about working out, which in turn was making her feel ashamed of the way her body looked. "I feel broken," she said, "and I feel like my husband will never love me the same way again."

"I have just the person for you," I said. "Her name is Katie Gilin. She has a doctorate in physical therapy and she's an expert in everything to do with the pelvic floor muscles. I think she'll be able to help you."

During the examination, Katie noted that Maria had difficulty using her lower abdominals and lower back muscles, and also had difficulty using her spinal muscles to transfer her weight. It also became apparent that she unable to contract her pelvic floor muscles quickly or to contract and hold the muscles for any length of time. In addition, she had a tendency to hold her breath during physical activity—all of which was creating increased pressure on the pelvic floor.

"It's really important for you to maintain proper pressure within your abdomen to decrease pressure on the pelvic floor, so strengthening your pelvic floor muscles will let you manage urinary leaking during activities," Katie told Maria. "There are also certain ways to learn to breathe that you can use while lifting things, and during other physical activities, which will help with your lower back pain."

Katie started Maria on a course of pelvic floor physical therapy, with core stabilization exercises to practice at home. Maria also used the biofeedback machine to visually see how to control her pelvic floor muscles, and how she could apply that control during intimacy with her husband

After eight visits of physical therapy, Maria reported to Katie and me that she had been able to be intimate without any urinary leaking and had gone back to jogging and weightlifting without fear of leaking.

"I thought I would have to wear a pad forever," Maria admitted to me. "I was so afraid of losing touch with my husband because of this. I'm going to tell all my friends about my experience with gaining back my confidence and true self, all thanks to physical therapy!"

While illness presents a struggle to the bond that exists in our relationships, overcoming struggles often creates even stronger bonds. Certainly, comforting one another after an illness is challenging, and role shifts can occur. Grief, loss, anger, and depression may be just some of the emotions that both partners must face. A team approach by healthcare providers is generally the most successful way to help a couple regain and maintain sexual health.

For example, healthcare specialties that work together to help couples maintain intimacy would include sexual health medicine, gynecologic care, physical therapy, psychopharmacology, and psychotherapy.

Coping strategies that helped couples in the prostatectomy study cited above included:
- being optimistic
- using humor
- reframing the experience in the larger context of beating cancer
- the strength of the relationship
- acceptance of low sexual function
- affection
- patience
- communication about sexual losses/changes
- the man's participation in sexual rehabilitation activities
- the partner's sexual interest
- regular sexual activity and willingness to experiment sexually
- using sexual aids

"We discovered that couples' capacity to recover

sexual intimacy was modified by their pre-existing strengths and vulnerabilities, their capacity to communicate about grief and mourning together and their ability to use positive coping strategies." (Wittmann et al, 2015)

Dating and relationships blogger Eileen Davidson, who was diagnosed with rheumatoid arthritis at age 29, says it's not all bad news. "For the few who can see past my illness, I am still just like anyone else—with some unexpected bonus traits." Among these, she notes that she's mentally strong, eats healthy and stays active, and has VIP parking thanks to her handicapped parking pass. "A little adversity hasn't held me back from living a productive life," she says to a prospective partner. "Why should it hold you back from being part of mine?" (CreakyJoints.org, 2020)

"I think a hero is an ordinary individual who finds strength to persevere and endure in spite of overwhelming obstacles," said actor and philanthropist Christopher Reeve; and in fact, Reeve and his wife, Dana, were inspirational in their public displays of affection, both before and after the accident that caused his quadriplegia.

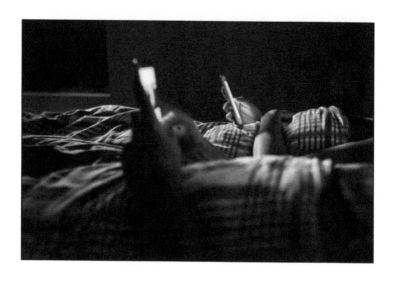

Myth #4: Good Sex Just Happens

"Instead of approaching sex as a natural, necessary, physical act, consider approaching it as a gift—an interest and an ability that can be cultivated. ... You won't have a great sex life unless you make it a priority to actually work on intimacy together."—Juli Slattery, 2009

Mind-blowing sex may be the norm in movies, but in real life, sex that is fulfilling for both parties isn't always a given.

The Sexual Advice Association fact sheet on lack of sexual desire and/or arousal describes the sexual response cycle as a three-stage process of desire, arousal, and orgasm, while noting that this may not be so straightforward in women: "Many women do not move through these stages in a step-wise manner (for example, some women may become sexually aroused and achieve orgasm as a result of a partner's sexual interest, but did not feel sexual desire beforehand). And some women may not experience all the stages (for example, they may experience desire and arousal but not orgasm)."

The fact sheet also notes that sexual desire and arousal can be negatively affected by physical or psychological issues (and often it's a combination of these issues). Depression, anxiety, relationship problems, sexual dysfunction in the partner, low self-esteem, and negative body image are among the psychological issues that are mentioned. However, sometimes the best advice is to seek professional guidance from a trained psychologist or psychiatrist. (sexualadviceassociation.co.uk, 2018)

It's worthwhile to reflect that women and men are not the same when it comes to readiness for sex.

As Kathy Koenigsknecht, a Pure Romance dealer who is getting her certification as a sex therapist, puts it: "Women are like crockpots: we take time to warm up. Men are like microwaves."

In my lectures, I tell the audience that men need about 30 seconds to decide sex sounds good and women need about 30 minutes of foreplay to be relaxed enough to be able to have an orgasm. That gets a laugh, and then I talk about "the nothing box."

The "nothing box" is what men use to free their minds for sex. It ensures that they're thinking of nothing during sex but sex. If nothing else is on your mind, then you tend to give your attention fully to what's happening to your body (and your partner's body). That's ideal during lovemaking.

Women don't have a "nothing box." In women's

minds, everything is connected to everything, which means that women are constantly thinking, which makes it really difficult to concentrate on only one thing, even if that one thing is something as great as sex.

For just one example, in order to have an orgasm, one must focus on one thing only, and that is having an orgasm. If women are in their typical state of mind of thinking/planning/worrying about everything and everyone, not only will orgasm not be possible, but being fully present in the act of sex will be impossible too.

That's why the "cake and icing" analogy from Myth #2 is so useful—even a slice of cake is beneficial for the relationship and the strengthening of the relationship bond—the icing is optional!

Women especially tend to imagine themselves as masters of multi-tasking who can do many things at once and be efficiently using every bit of brain all of the time. But that can be an unwelcome trait during sex.

You can find out more about "the nothing box" from popular pastor, speaker, and author Mark Gungor, in his YouTube video titled, "Tale of Two Brains Full" (https://www.youtube.com/watch?v=814eR5K7KD8), starting at 16 min. 10 sec., and going on to about 29 min. 10 sec. Pastor Mark has more than one video on YouTube, but in this particular video session, one of the first things he says is: "Men are very simple. S. E. X. Simple." Pastor Mark's presentation will make you laugh, I promise!

One viewer of that video session left a comment that I want to share: "While men and women, on average, have different needs, it's important to know that a large chunk of men really really want the emotional intimacy too. Although this is more common in mature men, men who also realize the emotional side is important too. Do not confuse age with maturity, they are only loosely linked." (YouTube.com, 2010)

For some, predictability leads to a sense of security. For others, adventure is the spice of life. Most of us fall somewhere in between: We like the security of knowing how things are going to be, but we don't mind the thought of exploring new things. Each person in a relationship won't necessarily be in the same place on this continuum, but that doesn't mean they won't be open to trying new things.

Mike was in my office for his RA checkup. He said things were going well with his joints and medications. He was exercising and taking great care of himself, so we had an extra ten minutes during his visit. I took the time to ask Mike about his wife, Sue, and their relationship.

He said, "Same old, same old—like bologna on white bread."

I couldn't help but ask him what he meant by that.

"I mean our relationship has become predictable and boring."

"Do you mean that your sex life is boring?" I pressed him.

"Yes!" he said emphatically.

He proceeded to describe their sex life: always at the same time on Saturday nights, always using the same position.

I asked what he had done to try to spice things up.

"Well, early on in our relationship I brought home a dirty movie for us to watch together, and Sue got upset that I'd gone to one of those sex shops without her, so I never tried that again."

"Aha!" I said, and I guided him through a conversation of how he could include Sue into trying something new with him. Then I asked him if he knew what Sue's "love language" was, and he said had no idea.

"Why don't you ask her over a romantic dinner out? Because if you fill up her love tank more often, she'll probably reciprocate with more sex and even trying some new ideas."

He wanted to give it a try.

Three months later Mike came in for his RA checkup appointment. I went into the exam room and Mike was not alone—he had brought Sue with him.

Sue said, "I wanted to meet you and thank you for talking to Mike. He's been acting differently at home and when I asked him why, he told me that his Nurse Practitioner had suggested he find out what my love language is, to help strengthen and build our marital bond. I've never heard him talk like that before!"

Sue shared with me that she had felt that their marriage was as good as it was going to be, and she had resigned herself to that—that she felt lucky to have a husband at all.

"But now, Mike is going out of his way to do nice things for me," she said, "and I'm feeling much more open to lovemaking and trying some new things. We're even planning a trip together, which we haven't done in years!"

"We're both excited about having new adventures together." Mike added, with a grin.

Lesson learned: It's never too late to try—to share—new things.

When dealing with loss of health and consequent physical challenges, it's especially important to keep the lines of communication open, to enjoy being together, and to try not to focus too much on preconceived ideas about how sex is supposed to be.

We can learn a lot from those who practice meditation, during which, in order to get to a higher level of consciousness, one must quiet the brain. As in meditation, during intimacy one can redirect the brain to focus on the senses: the scent of one's partner, the feeling of having one's skin touched, the heat of having another's body near yours, tastes, and the sight of your partner being intimate with you.

Being distracted during intimacy is one example of not being in the moment. When one is not fully involved 100% in the close bond of intimacy with one's partner, orgasm will often be an unachievable goal, and even enjoying the other acts of lovemaking can be difficult.

The Uncovering Intimacy website offers these 13 suggestions about how to be more "present" during sex:

1. Practice being mindful at other times.
2. Use meditative prayer.
3. Focus on the sensations.
4. Focus on what you and your spouse/partner are doing.
5. Try some "bedroom" talk.
6. Pay attention to your partner; try giving pleasure instead of receiving it.
7. Change what you're doing or change your position.
8. Reduce distractions (music off, tidy the bedroom ahead of time, etc.).

9. Focus on the visuals (watching yourselves in a mirror focuses the brain).
10. Take time to warm up to intimacy.
11. Take an active role in your togetherness.
12. Accept that your mind may wander — identify that stray thought and let it go.
13. Recognize what's happening in the here and now.

Enjoyable and mutually satisfying sex sometimes requires preparation. Partners should feel prepared both physically and emotionally. They should arrange a level of privacy that feels comfortable. Having a standing date can be a real help; for example, reserving one night a week to spend alone together. There are lots of ways to make sure that the intimacy won't be interrupted: ban attention-demanding electronic devices; confine pets to another part of the house or put them in the yard; arrange for children to be supervised elsewhere. Alternatively, go to a private location for a pre-arranged time period; hotel sex can be a real turn-on!

Readiness is especially important for individuals with physical complications or limitations. Those with joint pain and stiffness can benefit from a warm bath or shower prior to getting intimate (try it together!). Trying alternative positions, and using devices that enable different positions, can also help, as we will discuss in Myth #5.

Fatigue can also cause problems with intimacy, too. For instance, "first thing in the morning" sex may be good for some people when fatigue is an issue at night; on the other hand, morning sex may be uncomfortable or impossible if joint stiffness is a problem early in the day. Consider sex following a nap, or sex after the morning shower or bath.

Consider the sleeping arrangement, too—a king-size bed or two twins pushed together, gives each person more space, and can help the person with chronic pain find comfortable positions without unduly disturbing their partner.

One of my patients is Val, a 26-year-old mom with Crohn's disease. Val told me that she and her husband, Nate, make plans to spend time together for sex, but it seems like every time they're about to get intimate, her Crohn's symptoms flare up.

"I have to get up and run to the bathroom," she said. "Who can feel attractive with the bleeding and abdominal cramping and all the rest?"

One of my suggestions was that, when it happens, she and Nate could just snuggle, maybe spoon in bed, to help them stay close, and try for sex later on that day or evening, or the next morning.

Lesson learned: It might be a good idea for Val to keep a diary, in case the time of day, or something she had recently eaten or had to drink, was triggering the onset of symptoms at these times. It's also possible that the symptoms were being triggered for a psychological reason related to having sex; this, too, should be addressed.

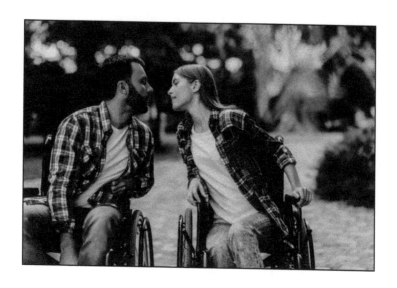

Myth #5: Disabled People Are Not Sexual

"Why begin a sex guide with what isn't true about sex and sexuality? Because wrong ideas about sex and disability affect us all."—*The Ultimate Guide to Sex and Disability: For All of Us Who Live with Disabilities, Chronic Pain, and Illness*, 2017

Whether or not one thinks of oneself as having a disability, society's mistaken beliefs do indeed matter, because disability and sex are not mutually exclusive.

"The taboos around disability and sex put limits on everyone ... Not only do they deny disabled people their right to a fulfilling sex life, they perpetuate rigid norms for the rest. [T]he truth (that most won't admit until they have to) is that illness and impairment are normal, everyday human experiences," writes Aly Fixter in *The Guardian*. "One in five people are disabled. Add people with health conditions that affect sex life (for example, erectile dysfunction), people who are adapting sex to their naturally ageing bodies and ... suddenly you're talking about a lot of people who don't fit the mold."

Aly goes on to quote activist Penny Pepper, who writes extensively about disability and sex, including in her erotica collection *Desires Reborn*, a collection of short stories that feature disabled people as the central protagonists in various sexual contexts.

"If disabled people aren't having sex, they would like to," says Penny. "And the reasons they're not are overwhelmingly to do with the barriers in society. I've known quite a few disabled people who [because of this] have resigned themselves to never having sex."

Penny adds, "If a non-disabled person says, 'Oh no, a disabled person can't have sex,' well, that really says more about that person's lack of imagination [than anything else]."

Aly suggests that a more accepting approach to the effects of disability and chronic illness on sex might include sex-related products and content made with the awareness that one-fifth of the audience may have a health issue that affects their sex life.

"Maybe we'd scrap 'sex tips' that guarantee orgasms or assume all bodies are alike and that penetration is the focus," she writes. "Maybe more non-disabled people would explore the idea of dating disabled people. And maybe it would enable more of us to accept our own imperfect, ever-changing bodies as they are, throughout our lives, and explore more sexual possibilities without shame—and a bit more imagination." (Fixter, 2019)

These are some other resources suggested in Aly's article:

- Leandra Vane, a sexuality blogger, book reviewer, and speaker who talks frankly about the challenges and joys of sex
- The disability-led charity Enhance the UK that offers online advice on sex and dating
- Canadian disability campaigner and writer Andrew Gurza, who created the hashtag #DisabledPeopleAreHot
- Popular influencers, such as the model Mama Cax and the retro fashion YouTuber Jessica Kellgren-Fozard, who celebrate disabled style, including customized mobility aids, while critiquing non-disabled beauty standards
- Imogen Fox, who offers frank posts and images about the realities of dealing with illness and bodily difference

A 23-year-old male wheelchair-user wrote to the syndicated sex advice column "Savage Love" to ask Dan Savage how he could indicate to women that he was interested in dating—that he was indeed a sexual being, not just a sexless person in a wheelchair.

Dan asked the authors of *The Ultimate Guide to Sex and Disability*—Miriam Kaufman, Cory Silverberg, and Fran Odette—to respond.

They wrote back: "Many people think 'paralyzed from the waist down' means 'turned into a block of ice down there.' [Non-paralyzed people] have been raised to believe that it isn't polite to ever ask a person with a disability anything about their disability, let alone about sex."

They went on to suggest that, on their first date, the young man and the young lady should watch *Murderball*, "a film about athletes in wheelchairs [that] has some fairly frank discussions about sex."

Aruma (a merger between House With No Steps, one of Australia's leading disability service providers, and The Tipping Foundation, a nonprofit community organization) counters common misconceptions about disability and sexuality with these 10 facts:

1. People with disabilities can be sexual and enjoy sex!
2. People with physical disabilities can have sex.
3. People with a disability are sexy.
4. People with a disability don't only have sex with one another.
5. Some people who use a wheelchair can still feel "down there."
6. Sex is not just all about each other's "privates."
7. People with a physical disability don't just "lie there."
8. People with a disability can and do use sex workers.
9. People with a disability can identify as LGBTQI [lesbian, gay, bisexual, transgender, transsexual, queer, intersex], too.
10. All people need to learn about and understand sex.

DeeDee came to see me for a routine checkup. She had

Ankylosing Spondylitis (AS) and had been my patient for years, but her AS had progressed to the point that she was using a wheelchair or walker due to pain and mobility options. After I reviewed with her the medications she was taking, we talked about her joint pain.

Then she said, "I have one more question for you."

"What's that?" I asked.

"It's a little embarrassing, but I promised Frida I would ask you," she said.

"You know you can ask me anything," I assured her.

She took a deep breath. "I'm having difficulty opening my legs open wide enough to have sex with Frida. Are there some exercises you can give me?"

I knew that she and Frida were a couple, so that didn't surprise me, but I didn't know how to help with this!

"I don't have a quick and easy solution right now," I admitted, "but give me a few weeks and I'm sure we can come up with something."

This complication was due to the fusion of DeeDee's sacroiliac joints, so I contacted a colleague who's a Doctor of Osteopathic Manipulative Medicine (DO) resident I've worked with before. He felt that osteopathic manipulation and a specific physical therapy program could help. I called DeeDee with the news and she was ready to get started.

After two months of intensive PT and OMM, DeeDee was able to regain some mobility in her sacroiliac joints—enough to allow for more satisfying intimacy with her wife.

At her next visit, I asked DeeDee how she was doing.

"You know," she said, "as soon as I stopped the home PT exercises and took a break from seeing the DO, my hips started to stiffen up again and intimacy became difficult again."

"Then you'll just have to keep yourself mobile in order to maintain your sex life!" I said.

She laughed and said she had to agree.

Lesson learned: This new knowledge and better understanding of her physical condition also encouraged DeeDee to use her walker more and her wheelchair less, to help maintain her joint flexibility.

Advances in technology are allowing people with mobility limitations and more profound injuries to participate in sexual experiences. For example, the Intimate Rider is a swing chair that allows the seated person to glide back and forth during intercourse; the FertiCare Personal is a hand-held vibrator that uses transcutaneous mechanical nerve stimulation; support slings and position aids help with positioning.

The Ultimate Guide to Sex and Disability: For All of Us Who Live with Disabilities, Chronic Pain, and Illness is probably the best and most informative book ever written on the subject of intimacy and disability. The authors describe how individuals with a range of disabilities have and maintain intimacy. There was such a positive response to the book that the authors started the Come As You Are Cooperative, a store in Toronto, Canada, that offers sex tools designed for ease of use for those living with disabilities. By adapting existing tools and designing new ones, they have created devices that work with different levels of sensation, mobility and motor control, as well as considerations for privacy (tools that are quiet and unobtrusive) and ease of cleaning. Products and extensive information are available online at https://www.comeasyouare.com. As they write in their book, "Sexual independence is an extremely potent form of empowerment."

Other devices, equipment, positioning products, and even furniture are available on a variety of online sites and stores. An excellent guide to what's available is *PleasurABLE sexual device manual for persons with disabilities* (and their partners). The booklet can be downloaded for free from various online sites; see Resource section.

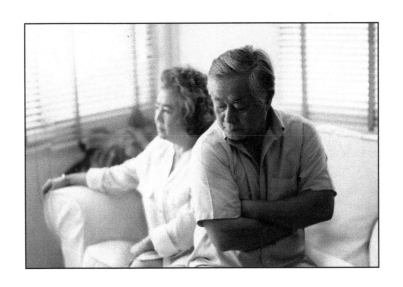

Myth #6: There Comes A Time When Sex Isn't Important

"The sexual relationship... is one of the most fundamental types of social relationships, and it has long been recognized as an essential part of human life."—Hui Liu et al, *The Journal of Health and Social Behavior*, September 2016

Some people believe sex is just for procreation, and that they should not enjoy sexual activities or engage in sex just for fun. We're not suggesting that anyone should be counseled to reject teachings of a lifetime, but it can be pointed out that sexuality is a normal part of being human: We were born with the ability to laugh, and digest, and move and think, and most of us were born with the ability to have an orgasm and enjoy pleasure. The body naturally releases dopamine in the brain in response to pleasure. In order to give ourselves permission to feel and experience sexual pleasure, we must normalize sexuality.

I recently had a patient say, "Well, we aren't trying to have any more children, so I don't really see the need for sex."

I replied, "In the animal kingdom sex is used for bonding and safety—if there's tension in the herd, then someone is going to be left behind, left hungry, or left unprotected. If everyone in the herd is relaxed, then no children are eaten! Sex is necessary in relationships to maintain bonding, keep the peace, and alleviate stress."

In a 2019 NBC News online article on sex and intimacy by Wendy Rose Gould, two psychologists explained why physical intimacy continues to be so important over time:

"Sex is important to the degree that it makes a couple happy," says Dr. Brian Jory, a relationship psychologist and author of *Cupid On Trial—What We Learn About Love When Loving Gets Tough*, "and the frequency and quality of sex that makes a couple happy varies greatly and depends on a lot of factors: their ages, values, lifestyle, innate sex drive, their health, and most of all, the quality of the relationship."

"Your relationship isn't going to fail just because the sexual aspect isn't as robust as it was many years (and perhaps several kids) ago," says Dr. Sanam Hafeez, a clinical psychologist based in New York City. "However, operating on autopilot without making a concerted effort to nurture physical intimacy can lead to decreased fulfillment, which is never good."

"Sex is important in a relationship. When we are looking at the brain and hormonal benefits, orgasm releases oxytocin which is the 'feel good' hormone that bonds us. This is why, when couples begin to feel that they are drifting or growing apart, they're mostly likely to report a lack of sex." (Gould 2019)

But don't think getting older is stopping single seniors from being sexually active—quite the opposite—and it's creating some very specific health issues, according to data from The Centers for Disease Control and Prevention on older Americans:

- Many widowed and divorced people are dating, but they may be less aware of their risks for HIV than younger people, believing HIV is not an issue for their age group, so they may be less likely to protect themselves.
- Women who no longer worry about becoming pregnant may be less likely to use a condom, thus less likely to practice safer sex. Yet age-related thinning and dryness of vaginal tissue may raise older women's risk for HIV infection.
- Although they visit their doctors more frequently, older people are less likely than younger people to discuss their sexual habits or drug use with their doctors—and doctors are less likely to ask their older patients about these issues.

Sex among seniors in retirement communities is also leading to increases in sexually transmitted infections (STIs), as reported in the *Orlando Sentinel*. In Arizona's Maricopa and Pima counties—home to large retirement communities just outside Phoenix—reported cases of syphilis and chlamydia were up 87% among those 55 and older in those counties, increasing twice as fast as the national average from 2005 to 2009.

In Central Florida, where retirement communities span several counties, reported cases of syphilis and chlamydia increased 71% among those 55 and older from 2005 to 2009, while South Florida saw a 60% increase in those two SDIs among the same age group, according to the Florida Department of Health. (Jameson, 2011)

Esther is a 67-year-old lady with lupus. She came to see me one day and said that she wanted to have intercourse with a man from church whom she'd been dating but wasn't sure she would be able to. I thought she was referring to her limited range of motion in her legs and hips. But it wasn't that—her concern was that she had never had intercourse; she was a virgin.

I asked, "When you were still having periods, were you ever able to put in a tampon?"

"No," she said, "that was always really tough."

"OK, I said, "before you even think about having intercourse we need to prepare your vagina," I showed her a vaginal dilator in a Pure Romance catalog I keep in the office, and told her, "You might want to consider this to help with penetration readiness, because you don't want your first experience to be incredibly painful." (I always recommend the Pure Romance company for sex aids, but there are other companies that sell these.)

Then we talked about how to combat vaginal dryness, which was an issue, and I also explained how she could improve her pelvic floor readiness by doing Kegel exercises regularly. Finally, I counseled her to discover through self-exploration what would arouse her and excite in her the desire for sexual activity—very important! And, as always, making sure her new partner was free of STIs would necessitate a frank discussion ahead of time.

Lesson learned: By including senior citizens in sexual health discussions, we make it easier for them to bring up any concerns, while also being able to confront any potential hazards.

At the other end of the age spectrum, of course, are children who are entering the world of sexual expression. They not only deserve but are desperate for accurate and compassionate guidance. A sex ed handbook for parents by Dr. Laura Berman presents information using easy-to-understand language by age group to help children understand their bodies, their emotions, and their responsibilities. The guide concludes:

"Sex isn't about taking, using or hurting—it's about giving and receiving pleasure, in a physically and emotionally safe manner. Make sure your daughter knows that when she is old enough to be sexual she should be receiving pleasure and not just giving it. Make sure your son knows he should be giving pleasure and not just taking it. Let them know that respect is the key to a happy, fulfilling sex life ..." (*The Sex Ed Handbook: A Comprehensive Guide for Parents*, 2015)

There are other components to relationships that can come as a surprise when we learn of them. A disturbance to a person's emotional connection with a partner will have an effect upon the relationship, too, regardless of age or gender.

Ann came to see me at the clinic with a complaint of low libido. I asked her how long this had been going on, and she replied that she had had trouble with low sex drive for about one year and it was really upsetting to her.

I pointed out that there are many possible reasons for a low sex drive, such as:

- Low level of DHEA—a hormone that allows our bodies to produce estrogen, testosterone, and progesterone
- Medications like antidepressants, anti-seizure medications, narcotics
- Stress, fatigue, and distractions
- Overall or specific issues with pain
- Thyroid dysfunction
- Low self-esteem/body image issues
- Fears of incontinence/pain during sex
- Trust and relationship issues

I said, "We can do some simple blood tests to evaluate for any physiologic causes of your low libido. Now, tell me about your relationship."

She proceeded to tell me that she absolutely hated her husband, who had cheated on her, and she used several explicit words to describe him.

I must have looked confused, so she added, "But I miss having sex."

Just to be sure I understood her, I asked, "With him?"

"Yeah," she said. "I hate him, but I still like to get off."

"OK," I said, "I understand. I can tell you that trusting and liking your partner usually improves libido, so I think it would help for you to talk about all this with someone who's trained to help you deal with these issues." I gave her a list of counselors to choose from and asked her to follow up with me after she'd had several counseling sessions.

Lesson learned: Sometimes you have to know when to refer out.

And, by the way, in February 2020, Tracey Cox, best-selling author of *Supersex for Life* (and 14 other books on sex and relationships) published her new book, *Great Sex Starts at 50: How to Age-Proof Your Libido*. Just a little reminder that there's no age limit on sex!

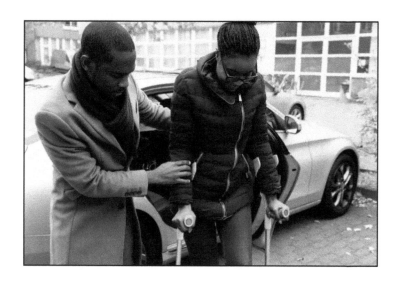

Myth #7: My Health and Physical Changes Have Made Me Unattractive

"Feeling you aren't attractive enough to be with your partner can be a very demoralizing and isolating experience."—relate.org.uk, 2018

We must not discount the impact that even the smallest loss of joint flexibility or outbreak of malar or psoriasis rash or joint swelling or even the inability to wear high heels can have on a person's self-esteem. These and so many other effects of illness can create a personal stigma—one that is often unfortunately reinforced by today's media and societal pressures. For example, weight is often an issue for people, because they believe that a particular body appearance creates a negative impact on their sexual attractiveness.

Many studies have been done that examine how one's body image can negatively affect one's ability to become aroused and one's subsequent sexual performance. In one, researchers in Ontario, Canada, used the Female Sexual Functioning Index to create a survey they administered to 88 sexually active women in heterosexual romantic relationships. The questions in the survey asked about body image and composition and sexual functioning.

The survey results indicated that dissatisfaction with one's body predicted a gradual loss of desire and arousal, as did the feeling that others also evaluated one's body negatively. Feeling negatively about one's appearance predicted a lessening in arousal. Negative thoughts and feelings about one's body during a sexual encounter (body image self-consciousness) predicted a lessening in both arousal and orgasm. (Quinn-Nilas, 2016)

When I was a student at Michigan State University in 1989, I took part in a study on body image that I still remember. The researchers separated the male and female participants—men in one room, women in another—and showed both groups identical pictures of various body types. We were then asked to rate which images we found the most sexually attractive and which images we thought the opposite sex would find the most attractive.

The results of the study showed that the men found the images of the fuller-figured women more sexually attractive—unlike the usual portrayals of stick-thin women as models and actors and other superstars. So, while it's important to be active and healthy, this study suggests that weight gain does not necessarily make a person unattractive.

Findings from these and related studies illuminate the importance of body image in sexual functioning, suggesting that strategies to improve body image could improve the sexual experience.

But just because who you are is much more important that what you are, physically, a physical change to one's body—even if it's invisible—can bring about a sense of negativity about oneself.

My patient, Emily, age 50, was complaining of pelvic pain during intercourse that became worse with orgasm. "The pain is an aching and burning during penetration, and stabbing and shooting pains whenever I have an orgasm," she said. "I feel like I'm not myself, and I'm embarrassed and ashamed to be avoiding all intimacy with my husband."

She said she also had a long-standing history of low back pain, especially on her left side that caused pain with prolonged sitting and standing. I decided the best thing to do was to refer her to a physical therapist, and sent her to Katie Gilin, DPT, who could address the back pain, which was affecting her everyday quality of life, and the pelvic pain issues.

Katie found that Emily's core and hip strength were weak, and also that she was not able to stabilize her pelvis during physical activities. Emily also had decreased coordination of the pressure system between her diaphragm and pelvic floor, and when Katie manipulated her pelvic floor muscles, Emily complained of both pelvic pain and lower back pain.

Katie and Emily decided on a treatment plan:

1. Exercises to improve flexibility, increase core and hip strength, and help her maintain proper pressure with breathing.
2. Manual therapy to decrease tissue tension to the back, adductors, and suprapubic region, and internal pelvic floor manual therapy to decrease tissue tension and promote relaxation. Emily agreed to explain the manual therapy techniques to her husband so they could use them at home.
3. Use of a pelvic floor wand massager.
4. Breathing techniques, and meditation and visualization strategies.
5. Sessions with a biofeedback machine to help retrain the hypertonic muscles that were likely creating the pelvic pain and irritating the nerve supplying the clitoris, causing the sharp pains during orgasm. The biofeedback device allows the patient to actually see the resting tone of the muscles and enables the use of relaxation strategies to make necessary adjustments.

Katie also suggested some alternate positions that would help Emily enjoy more comfortable intercourse and other aspects of intimacy with her husband.

"Warmup is important, too," she advised Emily, "just as it would be for any athletic endeavor, and don't forget to use a good lubricant!"

After 12 visits, Emily no longer felt pain with intimacy or orgasm, and her lower back felt much better. "Physical therapy was life-changing—my quality of life has really improved overall," she told me. "Plus, I thought I would

never have a 'normal' sex life with my husband again, and
I do!"

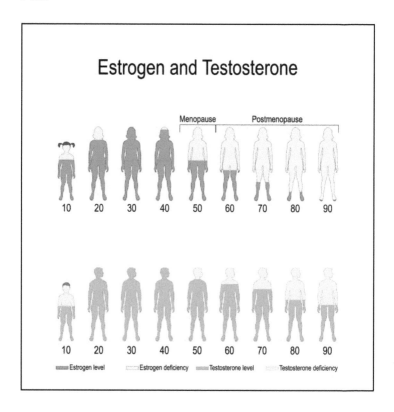

It is especially useful to understand that there are
certain changes in levels of estrogen and testosterone that
can lead to specific changes in sexual responses as we age.
    For women this can include:

- Lowered estrogen levels cause vaginal dryness, thinning and loss of elasticity in
  vaginal tissue.
- Slower arousal.
- Reduced intensity of orgasms.

- Some degree of urogenital atrophy may cause pain during intercourse.

For men this can include:
- Reduction in testosterone levels, which can diminish the ability to postpone ejaculation.
- More time needed to achieve an erection; erections do not last as long and are not as rigid.
- Less sensitivity in the penis.
- Less intense orgasms and longer time needed to achieve orgasm. (*Sexuality in Midlife and Beyond*, 2015)

On the AARP website, sex counselor and educator Michael Castleman writes that after age 50, men may begin to experience difficulty with ejaculation and orgasm. In Myth #2 we said that sex does not equal orgasm, and that's true. But nothing is more frustrating than being on the edge of that wonderful feeling, and not being able to get there! For a man, Castleman suggests identifying any factors that may be to blame:
- Getting older can weaken the pelvic floor muscles that trigger ejaculation; aging also can mean that the penis needs additional stimulation for ejaculation.
- Health conditions with neurological comlications, such as diabetes, multiple sclerosis, and spinal injuries, can affect the nerves that control orgasm.
- Alcohol use and medications, especially anti-depressants—but also drugs for anxiety, pain

relief, and blood pressure—can play a role in both erectile dysfunction and difficulty with ejaculation.

- Stress can be implicated if the man is experiencing negative emotions, such as anger, fear of getting a partner pregnant or contracting an STD, or conflicting ideas about sex and religious fundamentalism.
- Concentrating only on one's partner can interfere with orgasm and ejaculation if the man loses his own "erotic focus."

Mr. Castleman offers these suggestions that may help resolve difficulties, and can be useful for anyone regardless of gender:

- Rule out any possible infections.
- Determine if there are any issues with medications.
- Determine whether alcohol use is causing problems.
- Consider the effects of pain or nerve damage.
- Practice Kegel exercises to keep the pelvic floor muscles strong.
- Tell your partner about any favorite sexual situations.
- If intercourse is not providing enough stimulation for orgasm, ask your partner to help with manual or oral stimulation.
- Show your partner exactly what you like best (and also anything you don't like).
- Use deep breathing to relax the nervous system, which in turn helps erotic stimulation.

- Return to sexual fantasies that you've used in the past (and it's OK if they don't include your current partner).
- Use the right kind of personal lubricants to help increase sensitivity.
- Consider seeing a sex therapist, who can go in-depth to discover underlying issues that may be leading to sexual problems.
(AARP.org/relationships, 2019)

WebMD also offers a slideshow called "Exercises for Better Sex" (https://www.webmd.com/sex-relationships/ss/slideshow-better-sex-exercises) that includes suggestions to improve cardiovascular function, core strength, pelvic muscle strength, and flexibility. (A related slideshow, "Sex Drive-Killers" (https://www.webmd.com/sexual-conditions/ss/slideshow-sex-drive-killers) also makes some good points, albeit in general terms.)

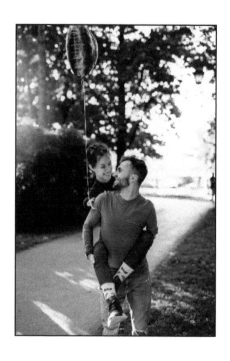

Myth #8: I Am Who I Am Sexually Because Of My Parts (Shape, Size, Etc.)

"I take off my one shirt, one shoe, pair of jeans. Try to hop to the bed and under the sheets before you can see. But you peel them back, and look, and smile. And then there are two bodies, a hundred kisses, one embrace, one surge of power and I lose count of everything. ... In the morning light, I see us in the mirror. Four arms, three legs, one stump, and your hand, resting there."—*Kissability*, 2014

I heard a sad story about a young woman who lost a fingertip in an accident. Her father was a friend of mine and he states his greatest grief was that the injury happened to the finger that her wedding ring would be worn on someday. I understood his pain, remembering how many pictures I have seen of individuals newly married holding hands and displaying their wedding rings as a symbol of the union of their marriage.

Loss of a fingertip, facial scars from discoid lupus, deformed knuckles from rheumatoid arthritis—all of these can impact self-esteem and create a personal stigma of illness. Likewise, the loss of any part of one's body, whether visible, like a leg or breast, or invisible, like a prostate or uterus, can be emotionally difficult and life-changing for the affected individual.

There are numerous studies, for example, that show that women feel less like sexual beings after a hysterectomy, mastectomy, or other gynecologic surgical procedure.

"The loss of an organ related to femininity, whether it is visible or not for others, refers to profound changes in the perception of self as part of the biological body [that] have direct influence on the social structure of the individual, in addition to its own functionality," note the authors of a study of Latin American women who had undergone various gynecologic surgeries in Rio de Janeiro, Brazil. "It is a loss that is reflected in the self-esteem, self-image, self-concept and elements that bring the feeling of being a woman." (Silva et al, 2016)

The Brazilian researchers offer several suggestions that can help when a person has undergone this kind of procedure.

- Try to see each patient as a person made up of many dimensions.
- Try to remember there are psychological and social contexts surrounding treatments and procedures.
- Try to understand the individual and sociocultural factors that interact to form the patient's understanding and experience of the surgical process.

"Knowing these meanings for her and the way she interprets what happened to her is an important tool for care. From this perspective, the nurse can be a key agent to help women find their own way to overcome the difficulties they face." (Silva et al, 2016)

The same is true for couples who face impotence after a man's prostate surgery: "We found that couples experienced not one, but two psychosocial transitions: cancer diagnosis is the first life-altering event, sexual changes after surgery are the second one." (Wittmann et al, 2015)

It wasn't so much grief as frustration that played a part in my home life not long ago. My 60-year-old husband, Chris, elected to have a procedure that would help with his symptoms of benign prostate hypertrophy (enlarged prostate gland, which can cause problems with urinary urgency, frequency, and flow), for which he had taken medications for years.

This was supposed to be a simple outpatient procedure—but there were complications. Not only did he had to keep the catheter in for a month instead of a week, but he continued to leak urine and had to self-catheterize; he had to use incontinence shields and guards; and worst of all, he was passing blood clots and in considerable pain. Chris was super frustrated that the surgical outcome had not gone at all as planned.

Six weeks went by this way, and he told me he was going to put the indwelling catheter back in place. He was tired of having to self-catheterize several times a day, dismayed at the skin breakdown he was experiencing, and nearly out of hope.

I had an idea. I suggested that he allow me to manually stimulate him to see if we could increase the blood flow to his penis and help with the healing.

He initially wanted no part of it. Here's a proud man who was now bleeding daily and wearing an adult diaper. He had lost his patience and much of his privacy. And his urologist had said absolutely nothing about resuming sex, as he was supposed to be healed in one week and we were now at six weeks post operation!

"Let's just try it for one week," I said gently.

He thought it over, considered the alternative, and resigned himself to the experiment.

Every other day manual therapy was performed, and within the week, my husband noted that the clots were reduced, and he was not having to catheterize himself every time he had to urinate. Within two weeks he was back to his old self and his skin breakdown and urination was back to normal.

Lesson learned: Never underestimate the power of a good hand job to restore blood flow and regain control of one's prostate health!

The Navy and Marine Corp Public Health Center's WII (Wounded, Ill, or Injured) Relationships and Intimacy Toolbox has valuable online resources for anyone who has been affected by an injury or change in appearance that is causing anxiety, concern, or fear. In particular, the "Dare to CARE" worksheet (see Resource list for website URL) offers these four strategies for communicating intimacy concerns to a partner:

- Capture your intimacy concerns by listing them in writing;
- Add a meeting with your partner to your schedule;
- Relate your concerns to your partner; and
- Engage your partner for feedback.

The Aging with a Disability Factsheet Series includes "How to Bounce Back" that defines the term "resilience" as "our ability to bounce back and keep going after a stressful experience." When people with disabilities were asked to describe resilience in their own words, these were some of the definitions they gave:

- Bouncing back or being "buoyant."
- "Rolling with" or "dancing with" a disability.
- Taking things one day at a time, while also planning for the future.
- Finding a "new normal" as life changes.
- Making the best of life with a disability.
- Trusting that stressful times will pass, like the weather.

In "Changes in Resilience Predict Function in Adults With Physical Disabilities," researchers discovered that increased resilience can lead to improved mood, less fatigue, better sleep, and improved physical functioning, and gave suggestions:

- Mindfulness meditation can help reduce stress and improve your sleep.
- Physical activity can help reduce stress and improve physical health.
- Building a strong social network can also help reduce stress and provide support for difficult situations.
- Counseling, such as cognitive-behavioral therapy, can help you manage emotions and thoughts in difficult situations. (Edwards et al, 2016)

While in no way meaning to diminish the very real feelings of anyone who feels they have become less than complete, we will add that, when partners of breast cancer patients are asked what they (the partners) care most about, the answer is so simple: they care that their loved one is alive and feeling well. The fact that there has been a loss or change in one or both of the breasts loses most of its meaning in contrast. "I don't care what they take from you as long as I can see your face" is a common remark.

"Most caring partners (both men and women) see their lovers as having many parts to love, and as being more than the sum of those parts." (You and Your Partner; breastcancer.org, 2016)

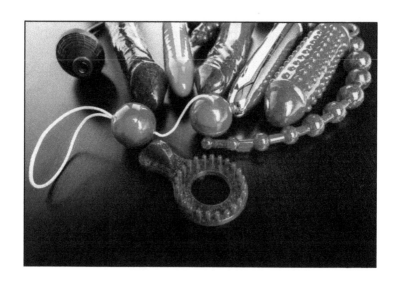

Myth #9: The Use of Sexual Aids Is Not Sexy

"A health issue doesn't mean your sex life will have to stop! Incorporating sex aids into your relationships means you don't have to give up on your sex life; you can discover more ways to enjoy sexual intimacy and pleasure either for solo play or with a partner."—JoDevine.com, retailer and sex education website

"A common misconception that 'proper' sex requires intercourse can leave some couples feeling frustrated if they are not able to have full penetrative sex due to physical disability, medical conditions, pregnancy, post-surgery after or during cancer treatments, side effects from medication, injury, or menstruation," writes Samantha Evans on the sexual health and education website Jo Devine, based in the UK. "Sex without intercourse can allow many couples to enjoy a more fulfilling sex life. With intercourse off the menu, this is where many sex aids come into play, offering sexual stimulation and sensations beyond mutual masturbation and oral sex."

Ms. Evans has a nursing background and, as you can imagine, I agree with her wholeheartedly! If you think sex toys are too much of a stretch for you or your partner, think about it this way: Most of us have heard of OXO—the company that designs solutions for cooking, cleaning, home organization, and more. This is their philosophy: "At OXO, we look at everyday objects and activities and we see ways to make things simpler, easier, more thoughtfully designed — better." Using gadgets and tools with ergonomic designs helps preserve our joints and makes our daily tasks easier. Why not look at sexual health aids the same way?

Another retailer and education source I recommend is the Come As You Are Cooperative, in Toronto, Canada (started by the folks who wrote the 2007 book, *The Ultimate Guide to Sex and Disability: For All of Us Who Live with Disabilities, Chronic Pain, and Illness*). The online store offers a wide assortment of toys, books, gear, and more, including products designed by and for people who are differently-abled. In "Learn How to Choose Your First Sex Toy" they offer an introduction to newbies: "With so much selection, choosing your first toy can be a daunting task. We've got suggestions for how to choose a vibrator, dildo, and strap-on harness, but before we get to those, there are three general key considerations: function, look and feel, and price." The article goes on to explain each of these factors in a bit more detail.

Good Vibrations, a "sex-positive sexual health and wellness toy retailer" (they also have gear, books, and movies) opened its first San Francisco store in 1977, and today their online store includes a ton of great articles, too, as well as an advice column helmed by award-winning author, activist, and sex educator Dr. Carol Queen.

An excellent source of products and information is the Pure Romance company, started by Patty Brisben with the goal of educating women about their sexual health. Patty used collaborative research from the Kinsey Institute at Indiana University to create products that are safe for women to use.

THE HISTORY OF THE VIBRATOR: A TIMELINE

The Early 1880s
British doctor Joseph Mortimer Granville invents the vibrator as a medical device for men, primarily to treat pain, spinal disease, and deafness. The only use that might be considered sexual is vibrating the perineum as a treatment for impotence.[1]

The early 1900s
Various brands and styles of vibrators are marketed, as domestic and medical appliances, to the general public—men and women.[1]

1968
The Hitachi Magic Wand® makes its debut on April 25.[2]

Mid-1970s
Artist, feminist, and sex educator Betty Dodson begins offering Bodysex Workshops that instruct women on using vibrators for masturbation, and in 1974 publishes her first book, *Liberating*

Masturbation: A Meditation on Selflove.[3]

1977
Good Vibrations, a "sex-positive" sexual health and wellness retailer of vibrators, sex toys, and more, opens its first store in San Francisco, California.[4]

1997
The worker-owned cooperative, Come As You Are, opens in Toronto, Canada selling vibrators and other sex toys, lubricants, books, DVDs , and products designed by people who are differently-abled.[5]

1999
Historian Rachel Maines publishes her book, *The Technology of Orgasm*, which is responsible for the unproven belief that vibrators were designed to help male doctors relieve women patients' "hysteria" with orgasm.[6]

2010
Sarah Ruhl's 2009 play, *In the Next Room (or the vibrator play)* is nominated for the Tony Award for Best Play and is a finalist for the Pulitzer Prize for Drama. The play is "an inventive work that mixes comedy and drama as it examines the medical practice of a 19th century American doctor and confronts questions of female sexuality and emancipation."[7]

Sources:
[1] Hallie Lieberman, "(Almost) Everything You Know About the Invention of the Vibrator Is Wrong," *The New York Times*, January 23, 2020
[2] Christopher Trout, "The 46-year-old sex toy Hitachi won't talk about," *Endgadget*, August 27, 2014
[3] Personal communication with Carlin Ross, Esq., Betty A. Dodson Foundation, August 17, 2020
[4] Good Vibrations online store, https://www.goodvibes.com/s/
[5] Come As You Are Cooperative, https://www.comeasyouare.com/
[6] Robinson Meyer and Ashley Fetters, "Victorian-Era Orgasms and the Crisis of Peer Review," *The Atlantic*, September 6, 2018
[7] The Pulitzer Prizes, https://www.pulitzer.org/finalists/sarah-ruhl-0

Does it surprise you to learn that the number one sexual aid is lubricant? We often don't think of lubricant as a tool, but sex without lubrication can be painful or impossible. There are many lubricants on the market, and it can be confusing to determine the pros and cons of each, because there are so many issues to consider. And don't confuse lubricants with moisturizers. Although the Food and Drug Administration does not require labeling that clearly indicates the differences, lubricants and moisturizers are not interchangeable! Dr. Lynn Wang, a practicing gynecologist with Main Line Health Physician Partners in Wynnewood, Pennsylvania, shares this information from her handout, "Lubricants 101," which you'll find in Appendix A.

As we complete this book, in July of 2020, the pandemic of the COVID-19 virus is causing illness, death, and uncertainty throughout the world. Most of the U.S. has been practicing some form of physical distancing since March, lots of businesses remain closed, and telemedicine visits are becoming increasingly common. Interestingly, I've found that the intimacy—but at the same time the feeling of distance—of telemedicine has allowed my patients to be more open about some confusing and embarrassing issues. These issues do take time to discuss, sort out, and resolve; I hope these "virtual" office visits will make it easier for patients to ask me for help.

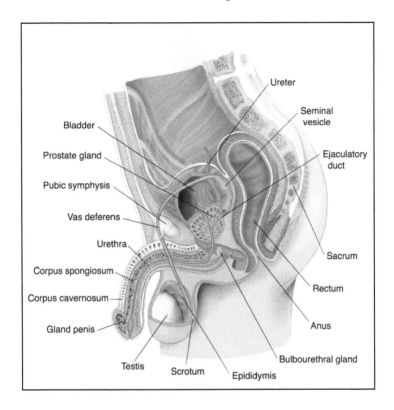

During a telemedicine visit with Edger, age 56, who has Ankylosing Spondylitis, he told me that he felt his treatment was not as effective as it once was. He also said that his back pain had worsened and he was having more foot and ankle pain.

"And I'm having another problem," he added. "This is probably not your field and I'm not sure if you can help me ..." He paused, and I got it.

I said, "Are your man parts still working?"

"That's the issue," he said, sounding anxious. "I can't talk to my Primary Care nurse—she's, like, 25, and I doubt she'd even know what to tell me anyway."

I instantly reassured him that this is quite common in

AS and, in fact, is often one of the first reasons men with undiagnosed AS go to the doctor: The spinal nerves help the penis to function, so anything affecting the spinal nerves can cause problems related to impotence.

I pushed further and asked, "What about morning erections? Are you still getting those?"

"Sometimes, but not always," he said, "and they're not what they used to be."

"What about intercourse?"

"Well, I try, but I'm just not firm enough to do anything."

I asked Edger if he had discussed this problem with his wife, Sarita, and he told me that the delayed ejaculation and the lack of firmness with his erections had become frustrating for them both, and they were avoiding sex.

"Excellent!" I said.

"What? Well, not for me!" he replied.

"No, of course not," I said quickly. "What I mean is, this is an issue that I think we can fix."

I talked to Edger about Viagra or similar products. He said he had heard of these medications but had not ever been prescribed them or tried them. We decided that he would try Viagra® (sildenafil) because it was now generic, so it would be cheaper and would be covered by his insurance.

"But it's not as simple as taking the pill and expecting an instant fix," I told him. "Many men try sildenafil and when they don't get an instant result the first time, they give up. Healthcare providers call this 'the first pass effect' because the first time you take a drug, your body processes it in a way that isn't very effective, and you might only absorb a little bit of the medication.

"Also, you have to take it on an empty stomach—no food, no alcohol!" I added. "Lots of guys take a pill and then take their partner to dinner and drink alcohol and too late they find that the drug doesn't work! You're better off having morning sex or sex before your date for the optimum efficacy. So—what did I just say?"

Edger smiled and said, "Viagra will work best ON AN EMPTY stomach!"

"Yes!" I said. "I'm going to prescribe 100 mg tablets for you, which will allow you to take half a pill and get twice as much from the pharmacy. And you need to have a conversation with Sarita."

He disagreed. "I want to surprise her," he said.

"NO!" I nearly shouted. "That's exactly what you don't want to do."

"But why not?" he asked.

"You have to tell her that we had this conversation so she can prepare! Women in their 50s have vaginal dryness and changes to their bodies as well," I explained, "and you don't want to hurt her with your new firm erection, right? You need to take the time for plenty of foreplay, and she needs to have some good lubricant ready as well."

I encouraged Edger to try the Viagra first on his own. "But," I added, "a man can't just sit and wait for the erection to pop up—he has to stimulate himself manually to get an erection first, then allow the medication to sustain the erection. OK?"

He listened and seemed ready to try the medication. I told him that on his next visit we would revisit this issue to ensure this treatment was working for him, because, if he could get an erection but was still having issues with delayed ejaculation, we may want to try something else.

He agreed to the plan and so far, things are going better in the bedroom for both Edger and his wife!

Lesson learned: It's a disservice for a healthcare provider to write out a prescription for a medication that increases vasodilatation to the penis without first educating the person on how to properly use the drug. People can't be expected to magically know how to use medications, or not to try to use them after a full meal and alcohol. As healthcare providers and caring individuals, we must educate so that others can have satisfying intimacy.

And speaking of physical distancing ... What happens when there's a pandemic, and you and your main squeeze don't live together, or one of you has to stay isolated due to work or parenting commitments? This might be a good time to think about making technology really work for you! A standing date for good old-fashioned phone sex can help keep a long-distance relationship alive—while helping to relieve the stress of these uncertain times.

The sex toys and sex-positive education site Good Vibrations agrees: "Social distancing is definitely the move right now, but that doesn't mean your sex life has to take a hit. Whether you're isolating without your partner and are relying on phone calls, video chat, and endless messaging on insta, or are shooting your shot on Tinder or Lex, sexting and digital dirty talk can provide some sexy distracting from the news and can boost intimacy, even if you aren't in the same place as your partner!" (goodvibes.com, 2020)

And that brings us to a controversial subject:

Pornography.

What is pornography? Is it the same or different than eroticism? How do we know which is which? And what a place do they have in today's society and in our personal relationships?

The online Merriam-Webster Dictionary (MWD) gives three definitions of pornography: "1. the depiction of erotic behavior (as in pictures or writing) intended to cause sexual excitement; 2. material (such as books or a photograph) that depicts erotic behavior and is intended to cause sexual excitement; 3. the depiction of acts in a sensational manner so as to arouse a quick intense emotional reaction."

And the MWD definition of erotic? "Devoted to, or tending to arouse sexual love or desire."

Eroticism is as old as the proverbial hills. In fact, the artistic depiction of sexual acts has been around since prehistoric times: Cave drawings of pubic triangles, vulvas, and erect penises, and figures in sexual poses, have been found in deep cave rooms in ancient archeological dig sites.

Fast (really fast!) forward to the late 1960s, when pornographic movies and printed erotic literature became accessible and available for sale in public venues in the U.S. Yet there was a stigma attached: customers often had to slip into back alley sex shops to find magazines or sex toys, and have X-rated videos delivered by mail in unlabeled brown paper parcels.

In the 70s and 80s, small sex-shops and adult bookstores became more commonplace (although not always welcome in some neighborhoods), and pay-per-view cable television channels showed increasingly stimulating fare. And then came the 1990s, when the World Wide Web began, and (with its underground counterparts) enabled access to all sorts of erotic and pornographic materials in the privacy of our homes. Is that a good thing, or a bad thing, or a "when we need it" convenience?

I'm not saying that there's anything wrong with using sexual imagery to spice up your love life. After all, this easy access to porn and erotica, sex toys and paraphernalia to support all kinds of personal kinks has certainly created new possibilities and opened up much-needed horizons and conversations. But this instant access can sometimes have unhappy consequences.

One afternoon, Sarah came to the clinic for her fibromyalgia checkup. I asked her how she was doing.

"Fine," she said, in her usual flattened tone.

I asked her about her pain level and how she was managing her pain.

"I'm trying to get rest and exercise some," was her only comment.

When I waited to see if she had anything to add, she then admitted she was having headaches regularly and that she wasn't sleeping well.

"What about your home life?" I asked

"Things are good with my husband," was all she said, but I suspected there was more to what was going on with her.

I said with a smile, "You know, having sex regularly increases your pain threshold, and improves your sleep quality, too."

She looked at me and started to cry. I sat down next

to her and asked her what was wrong. She told me that William, her husband, spent hours in his office looking at porn online and masturbating.

"I don't understand why, when I confronted him and told him it was the same as cheating on me, he said he didn't agree," she went on. "He said if he was not seeking out other women to have sex with, then he was not breaking the sanctity of our marriage vows. I feel shut out of his sex life, and I resent the amount of time he spends looking at other naked women."

And then she added sadly, "He must find me unattractive if he has to use other women for his sexual desires."

I asked her how long this had been going on and she said she had found out a year ago but suspected it had been going on for years.

"He's spent a lot of money on porn subscriptions and movies, and I have no idea what to do about it," she said, crying.

I tried to explain that an addiction to pornography is like an addiction to gambling or illegal drugs or even sex. When someone views pornography, the brain releases a chemical called dopamine which makes them feel happy. Pornography creates a feedback loop by causing feelings of happiness and excitement at watching things that are naughty and satisfying oneself by masturbating. Once the high of watching the pornography ends and the dopamine chemical high wears off, an individual goes back to feeling normal.

"It's just like getting high on a drug," I told her. "When the euphoria of the drug wears off, often the person starts thinking about what they can do to get that 'high' feeling again."

I asked Sarah if she had seen a marital counselor with her husband or discussed doing so with him. She said William would never go to counseling as he would never want anyone to know about his personal business. "He told me he didn't understand why I was making such a big deal out of it; what he did was not hurting me or the relationship, in his opinion."

I asked Sarah if she might try going to a counselor by herself, to see if that could help with her self-esteem. I gave her some suggestions on how to communicate better with William and mentioned that a counselor or therapist would be able to help her learn communication skills as well.

I also gave Sarah the name of a book I thought would be especially helpful to her and William. It's called *Laugh Your Way to a Better Marriage*, written by Mark Gungor, a pastor, motivational speaker and writer who has more than 30 years of experience sharing principles for marriage that empower couples without being "preachy." Mark talks about how pornography objectifies women into breasts and vaginas. He also explains to husbands that, to honor your wife, you must look at her as not sexual parts, but rather as the person who has been by your side and has years of shared experiences with you. He guides couples along the journey of respect and honor for one's spouse through regular sex with each other, and he explains how using that will boost the bond that fuels the marriage. The 2009 book is based on his weekend seminar, which has also been made into a four-DVD set.

Lesson learned: Erotica of all kinds can be used as a sex aid. Just look at the success of the book *50 Shades of*

Gray (2011), which I always think of as the first soft porn targeted to women. Women already had romance novels, but we weren't being very open about how the writing made us feel sexy; and then this came out and everyone was talking about it out loud. I think that the more women are cued to talk about sex, the more they're going to think about their own sexuality. From there it's just a small step to engaging in sex.

Overall I believe that a relationship will probably prosper from experiencing erotica together. In other words: Let your partner know about your turn-ons; it's the best way to discover what you can do together. There's no need to deny or give up your fantasies! But sharing can be rewarding, too, in many ways.

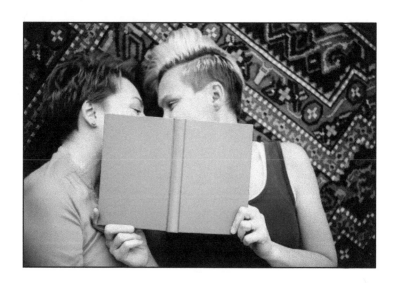

Myth #10: There's Nothing More I Can Learn About Sex

"You can bottle up your sex-related questions or ask your idiot friends. Or, you can call up ... experts for sex advice on their one surefire trick in the bedroom."—Judy McGuire, 2018

Ms. McGuire goes on to interview experts for her Esquire.com article, "Experts Tell Us 13 Ways to Have the Best Sex Ever." Topics covered include the importance of learning how to control your breathing; how long intercourse ideally lasts; hints about performing and receiving oral sex; how to watch porn with a partner; and how to stimulate a woman's G-spot.

Did some of those subjects surprise you?

After all, humans are lifelong learners. As our health

and relationships change and evolve, we too must change and evolve. Sex education isn't just a course we take in junior high school—learning about our bodies, our anatomy, and our relationships is a lifelong journey.

Karen was 22 when she came to see me about pain she was experiencing during intercourse. I asked her if the pain was new and she said it had begun with a new partner and happened with penetration. I assured her that there were lots of options and she agreed to see the Ob/Gyn first to rule out infection or sexually transmitted infections (STIs) or any other obvious issues. Young and old alike can get STIs, so those must be considered, along with any change in odor or pain or drainage. She agreed.

When Karen came back to see me and I asked her how her Ob/Gyn appointment went, she smiled and said, "It was crazy—the nurse practitioner was doing my pelvic exam and I told her I was having pain with penetration and she said she knew exactly what the problem was."

Karen said she was surprised, because she had already asked her primary care doctor and had been having symptoms of pain with penetration for six months, with no answers.

Then she looked at me and grinned and said, "The problem is simple: I'm short."

Puzzled, I asked, "Yes, but what does that have to do with pain during intercourse?"

Karen laughed and said, "My vagina is short too, so every time my boyfriend thrusts into me he's banging into my cervix!"

She told me that the Ob/Gyn NP had suggested some position changes and, *voilà*, the pain was gone. She added that her boyfriend now knows how to be careful, and they created a "safe word" so that, if a particular position was painful for her, she could signal a need for a position change so as not to have pain with her pleasure.

Lesson learned: One of my favorites—Never miss the obvious!

No discussion on new information would be complete without mentioning recent advances in virtual reality (VR) sex and in the manufacture of sex robots.

A *Newsweek* "Tech & Science" article from December 2018 predicts that "by 2025, the virtual reality (VR) adult-entertainment business will be worth around $1 billion—making it the third largest entertainment industry after video games and the NFL. ... Gadgets such as VR headsets, synched vibration of intimate parts and sex toys can help to make the whole experience as 'real' as possible."

Sex robots, too, are becoming both more advanced and more affordable, able to speak and react both sensually and verbally.

Not everyone considers these tech offerings as a positive development. In an op-ed piece published in *The New York Times* in July 2017, Laura Bates wrote, "By making these robots as realistic as possible—from self-warming models to those that speak and suck, from some with a pulse to others that flirt with their owners—their creators are ... effectively reproducing real women, complete with everything, except autonomy."

Bates is the founder of the Everyday Sexism Project, an online catalog of stories of gender inequality from around the world, and the author of the 2017 book, *Girl Up*, a feminist field guide for today's young women.

A different point of view comes from Hallie Lieberman, in her March 2018 post, "In Defense of Sex Robots": "By using them to teach consent, guide our partners to better satisfy us, and then use them to better satisfy ourselves, we can welcome them into our bedrooms. Sex robots don't have to be our enemies: They can be our partners instead." Lieberman is a historian of sex and sexuality and author of the 2017 book *Buzz: A Stimulating History of the Sex Toy*.

Whatever your personal opinion, it will help to keep an open mind when talking to your partner about these topics.

If sexual interest or response isn't as it once was—whether following breast cancer or other surgery or procedure, or a chronic illness diagnosis—a head-to-toe massage can help to turn things around. The "Beyond Intercourse" fact sheet suggests that "Massage is a wonderful relaxant and an aphrodisiac. Give it a whirl, music and body oils included." Providing stimulation by hand using a lubricant can also be gratifying as each partner relearns and discovers more about what pleases the other person, and themselves. (breastcancer.org, 2017)

Probably nothing makes people feel less like being intimate than pain. And for many people with chronic health conditions or illnesses, pain is a constant.

Pain during intercourse can be due to various emotional or physical factors, and we strongly encourage anyone with long-lasting pain to seek treatment so that their intimate experiences are more enjoyable. But there are lots of non-sexual ways, too, to maintain intimacy with a partner: holding hands while taking a walk, having a candle-lit dinner for two, or watching a romantic movie snuggled up on the sofa are just a few.

A lot of my women patients say, "It just hurts to have my partner touch me."

"Well, could you tolerate two minutes of back massage?" I ask.

"Yeah, I guess I could do that," is the usual reply.

"OK, then," I say, "if you can stand for your partner to massage your back for two minutes, then one thing's going to lead to another. You can shake hands and agree to start there."

And you know what? They laugh, and go home and try it, and a connection is made.

One of the best exercises I can recommend is the Kegel exercise—a contraction of the pelvic floor muscles. It was developed by Dr. Arnold Kegel in the late 1940s for women who had lost some bladder control after giving birth.

The fact sheet "Pelvic Floor Health for Women" from SexualityResources.com explains, "The pelvic floor consists of 14 different muscles, arranged in three layers, that form a supportive sling in the lower pelvis. In a woman's body, the pelvic floor muscles surround the urethra, vaginal opening, and anus."

These muscles do more than keep the pelvic organs in place and the pelvic bones stable—strengthening the pelvic floor, as you have read previously, can improve sex:

- The pleasurable muscle contractions felt in the genitals during orgasm are due to strong pelvic floor muscles.
- Orgasms that feel bigger and stronger when

the pelvic floor muscles are strong.

- Good flexibility in the pelvic floor muscles allows more comfortable vaginal penetration.
- Strong pelvic floor muscles help keep urine inside the bladder at moments of unexpected belly pressure (laughing, coughing, lifting, sneezing, jumping), and help keep stool inside the rectum until the pelvic floor is consciously relaxed to allow it to pass.

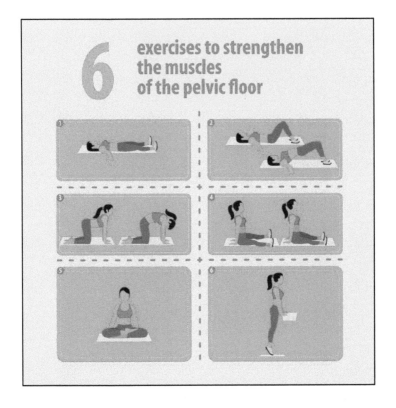

6 exercises to strengthen the muscles of the pelvic floor

For women, performing Kegels prior to getting intimate stimulates blood flow in the vaginal region, which helps prepare the area physically; but the very act of doing the exercises also helps to prepare the mind for the pleasures of sexual activity.

But Kegels are an equal-opportunity exercise: Studies have shown that a strong pelvic floor helps to improve erectile function, control ejaculation, and intensify orgasm for men as well! (Siegel, 2014)

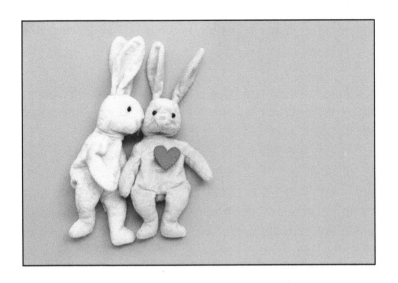

What Does "Honor Your Partner" Mean?

Part of having a great sex life is honoring your partner. We have already spoken of Gary Chapman's book, *The Five Love Languages*, and the absolute importance of figuring out your partner's "love language" so you can "fill up their tank" regularly.

Another way to honor your partner is to respect how they are different from you. We're often attracted to someone because they're different or exciting; but as the relationship evolves, we often want them to think or feel or act like we do. It goes back to that saying: "I love you so much—now change."

I realized the importance of this in my own life. I am very attracted to the man who is now my second husband—I think he looks, and behaves, like Robert

DeNiro. Chris is a noticeably confident man. He has an air about him that, no matter what happens, he has everything under control. He has amazing protective instincts and always makes me feel safe. He is also very much a gentleman—among the many ways he shows how he feels about me is by opening the door for me, including my car door, every day.

Falling in love with this man was extremely easy. Respecting who he is has been a challenge. You see, in my first marriage, yelling was the most common form of communication between me and "Paul." There was little trust on either side and no desire to improve communication.

Everything is different in my marriage with Chris. Early in our relationship, when Chris and I would disagree, I would raise my voice. I soon realized that this tactic was NOT going to work with MY Robert DeNiro. Chris is my senior by 10 years and has his own way of doing things. He does not need any help driving, loading the dishwasher, folding 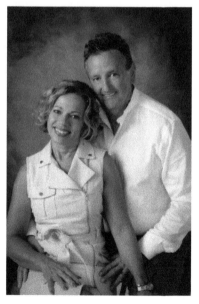 clothes, or fixing things around the house. He has taught me how important it is not to emasculate your partner. He commands respect—but he also reciprocates willingly by honoring me.

I've often thought that the process of taking away a person's sense of self starts after the birth of a child. Often, men (but sometimes women) have no experience with child-rearing. Thus, one partner assumes the care of the infant and starts directing the other partner how things should be done for the infant: how the bottles should be warmed up, how the diapers should be changed, how the infant likes to be rocked or talked to or burped, etc.

These decisions then spill over into how the house should be organized, how the money should be spent, how the groceries should be put away, and other aspects of the home until one spouse is running the show and the other spouse is taking orders. This can lead to resentment for both people: the one who's always making the decisions never feels rested and cared for; and the one who's always in the subordinate role loses the confidence to take charge, protect the family, and manage the household. This pattern can damage and ultimately kill a marriage.

I've also come to understand that my husband does not think like me. Not many people think like I do, but what's important to remember is that we're all individuals.

Chris and I were recently at a birthday party for my adult daughter Brittany. She's gay and is in a committed relationship, and there were many couples at the birthday party, both gay and straight. One of Brittany's friends was going around the room asking a party question: Would you want to have sex with a clone of yourself?

I quickly answered, "No way."

"Why not, Mom?" Brittany asked.

I explained that I knew how my parts work and how I looked and felt, and I like having sex with someone who is vastly different from myself. Chris agreed and said he would not be interested in having sex with a clone of himself, either.

I often think about that party question when I find myself wishing my husband would be more like me about something. When I get frustrated because he doesn't do the thing just like I do the thing, or because he moves at his own pace, or because he drives faster, slower, or different than I do, I think to myself: Would I want to be married to myself? And the answer is always "No!" I love him *because* he is different.

Over time I've learned to best honor my husband by respecting him and letting him handle things. When I get frustrated with him for not thinking or acting like I do, then I focus on WHY I fell in love with him in the first place.

Relationships are challenging and we are constantly learning how to be a partner. Respecting one's partner and their individuality and personality is key to maintaining stability in the relationship. Part of this relationship maintenance is having regular open communication. Communication is paramount for maintaining intimacy, having satisfying sex, and keeping the relationship healthy. You must be able to safely ask for what you need, and you must feel like you are being heard and respected in your wishes, without compromising your partner's needs.

Conclusion

There were several goals for this book: to shatter myths that hinder people from making and keeping intimate connections; to help readers feel more comfortable on the subject of sexual health; to help healthcare providers be better prepared to bring up the subject of sexual health with patients; and to provide real-life examples of how to talk with a partner about sex and intimacy.

I believe that each of us will be able to effectively communicate about sexual health, and feel more comfortable with the discussions, when we:

1. Bring up the subject of sexual health as part of the hierarchy of needs.
2. Approach each other as an individual, regardless of sexual preferences, sexual orientation, or gender identity.
3. Understand our own feelings about sex.
4. Remain open to an awareness of sexual activities that are unfamiliar.
5. Remain open to an awareness of religious and cultural customs and taboos around sex.
6. Broaden our own understanding of sexual health resources and referral possibilities.
7. Normalize the conversation with phrases like, "Many people experience this ..." and "As you may already know ..."
8. Use online search terms like "intimacy" and "sexual health and _____" rather than "sex and _____."

9. Never doubt that physically disabled people are interested in having sex.
10. Include the subject of safe sex.

In the words of the authors of *The Ultimate Guide to Sex and Disability*: "Sexual independence is an extremely potent form of empowerment." What more could we want for each other than that?

The Last Word(s)

We've examined a lot of ideas about sex, intimacy, and sexuality in this book. Some of this you may have known; some of it may be new to you. I hope what has been shared will help you give encouragement and hope, whether you use the information professionally or personally (or both!).

Overall, we believe four important points have emerged from the work presented here.

1. Our definition of sex will naturally change over time due to health issues or changes in desires.
2. Losing the ability to maintain an erection or tolerate penetration or reach orgasm does not make us any less sexual.
3. Sex is a shared form of intimacy—therefore, true intimacy is the goal of sex, and sexual expression will evolve out of necessity.
4. No matter which medical diagnosis or physical condition a person has, no one should have to give up sex or do without intimacy.

We'll leave you with this quote from one of the participants in the book *Kissability: People with Disabilities Talk About Sex, Love, and Relationships*. Her name is Constance. She was asked "What's better than sex?" Her answer: "Love is better than sex. Love and life."

Appendix A: Personal Lubricants

Dr. Lynn Wang, a practicing gynecologist with Main Line Health Physician Partners in Wynnewood, Pennsylvania, shares this information from her handout, "Lubricants 101."

Types of Lubricants

- Water-based lubricants are considered "all-purpose" because they can be safely used with all condoms and sex toys; cleanup is easy and products won't stain sheets or clothing. Because water-based lubes soak into the skin over time, reapplication may be necessary. (Examples: Natural Moisturizing Personal Lubricant from Blossom Organics and Sliquid H2O Original Water Based Lubricant).

- Oil-based lubricants are not recommended for two reasons: oils can break down latex and polyisoprene condoms; and oils can also leave a coating in the vagina or rectum that can trap bacteria and lead to infections. (Examples: YES OB Organic Plant Oil Natural Personal Lubricant, Petroleum jelly/Vaseline®, olive oil, mineral oil, vitamin E oil).

- Silicone-based lubricants will be more slippery than anything water-based and will last longer, but will be harder to clean up and usually cost more. These formulations are safe for use with all condoms but should not be used with silicone sex toys. (Example: Wet

Platinum Lubricant from Shibari).

- Hybrid lubricants are often a combination of both water and silicone, with elements of both. (Examples: BabeLube Silk Blend from Babeland and Sliquid Silk Hybrid Lubricant).

When selecting a personal lubricant, Dr. Wang says it's also important to consider:

- The pH—how acidic or alkaline a substance is. Substances are ranked on a scale of acidity from 0 to 14; more acidic solutions have lower pH, and more alkaline solutions have higher pH. Neutral solutions usually have a pH of 7. Normal vaginal pH is between 3.5 and 4.5, which is very acidic; menopause causes the vaginal environment to become basic.
- The osmolality—the concentration of particles in a fluid. Certain lubricants contain ingredients that cause high osmolality (i.e., glycerin and propylene glycol) that can damage vaginal and rectal tissue.
- The ingredients—some may be irritants to delicate tissue, some may cause an allergic reaction, some may degrade a condom, some may degrade a sex toy or device.

Dr. Myrtle Wilhite, medical advisor for A Woman's Touch (sexualityresources.com), suggests avoiding these ingredients:

  ○ Polyquaternium 7, 10 or 15 (a synthetic polymer)

- o Nonoxynol 9 (an oil-dissolving spermicide)
- o Menthol (used either as a "cooling" or sensation enhancer)
- o Lidocaine (a numbing product)
- o Capsaicin (usually found in warming, sensitizing, or "arousal-enhancing" lubes)
- o Chlorhexidine (preservative found in many medical lubricants)
- o Herbal extracts and raw, unprocessed aloe gel (can provoke allergic responses)
- o Glycerin (may act as a food source for yeast)

"There are thousands of personal lubricants on the market," says Dr. Myrtle, "so choosing the right one for your needs can be tough. Every person has different behaviors, different skin pH (acid/base balance), different tolerance to friction, different biologic environment, and different moisture needs. It's also hard, if not impossible, for manufacturers to formulate 'the right lube.'

Dr. Wilhite recommends lubricants that:

- Stay slippery to the touch. "Some playful folks like to keep a plant mister or a water pistol handy to revive a water-based lube when it dries out."
- Have a pH between 4.4 and 5.5 (which will be compatible with most skin types). "Oils are fine for external use, and some men find that self-pleasuring with an oil or cream creates a

slippery, cushiony experience. However, the vagina is a sensitive environment that cannot easily clean out oils, and so using them vaginally may cause irritation or infection."

- Are a water-base and silicone blend OR a silicone-only base. "If your toy is silicone and you want to use a silicone lubricant, know that silicone lubes can ruin the surface of silicone toys." She suggests covering the toy with a non-lubricated condom and then putting the silicone lube on the outside. "If you only use toys externally, experiment to see if you like the feeling of lube, or not. Also, petroleum-based oils (mineral or baby oil) break down latex products."
- Use a genital-compatible preservative.
- Are available in sample sizes (for testing and travel).
- Come in a pump-type dispenser (prevents bottle contamination).
- Have a reasonable cost.

Appendix B: Sexual Orientation Terminology

By Kirsten Schultz, MS

Sexual orientation is a wide range of sexual and/or romantic attractions (or lack thereof) to other people. Some people may be **heterosexual** while others are not— and those fall under the large LGBTQ+ umbrella. The acronym **LGBTQ+** stands for lesbian, gay, bisexual, transgender, queer, and more as indicated by the plus sign. It is used to refer to anyone who is either not heterosexual or not cisgender (see the next section).

- Amorplatonic: Someone who experiences romantic attraction to others but prefers being friends or engaging in friends-with-benefits behavior to having relationships.
- Androsexual: Someone who is sexually attracted to people who present more masculine (masc).
- Aromantic: Someone who does not experience romantic attraction.
- Asexual: Someone who doesn't experience sexual attraction or desire.
  - Grey Asexual: Someone who occasionally experiences sexual attraction, but not usually.
  - (Antonym) Allosexual: Someone who experiences sexual attraction.
- Bisexual: Someone who is attracted to two or more genders.

- o Bicurious: Someone interested in potentially experimenting with people of genders other than the ones with whom they're normally friends-with-benefits or attracted to.
- Ceterosexual/skoliosexual: Someone who is sexually attracted to people who have a more androgynous or gender-neutral look. Cetero- is more preferred, as skolio- refers to bent or not necessarily normal.
- Demiromantic: Someone who only experiences romantic attraction if they have an emotional connection to the other person involved.
- Demisexual: Someone who only experiences sexual attraction if they have an emotional connection to the other person involved.
- Friend with benefits (FWB): A friend with whom one has occasional sexual relations, without a commitment or dating arrangement.
- Gay: A man sexually attracted to other men or a woman sexually attracted to other women.
- Gynesexual: Someone who has a sexual attraction to people who present as more feminine or femmes.
- Heterosexual: A woman sexually attracted to a man or a man sexually attracted to a woman.
  - o Heteroflexible: Someone who generally is heterosexual but is interested in exploring sexual relationships outside of the heteronormative standard.
- Lesbian: A woman sexually attracted to other

women.

- Monogamous: A relationship where two people are dedicated to each other exclusively. This is the general societal view of marriage.
- Monosexual: Romantic or sexual attraction to only one gender.
- Pansexual: Sexual and/or romantic attraction to people regardless of their gender. This can also be seen as attraction to all genders.
- Platoniromantic: Someone who experiences friendship/platonic attraction and sexual/romantic attraction the same way.
- Polyamorous: This term refers to a relationship that involves multiple people with the knowledge and consent of all involved. You may hear this called ethical non-monogamy as well. This could mean being in an open relationship/marriage, swinging, and more. An important term for providers to know is **fluid-bonded**, a term for partners who do not use protection with each other but do with others.
- Polysexual: Someone who experiences attraction to some genders, but not all.
- Queer: This is often used to describe a person who falls under the LGBTQ+ umbrella, regardless of their gender or orientation. Note: This term used to be a slur, but has been reclaimed by people within the LGBTQ+ community. Still, that slur status stands, so please don't use this to describe a patient unless they've signaled that they're okay with

it. Many LGBTQ+ people identify as queer, which is partially a sociopolitical identification—for example, those who participated in the Stonewall Riots (June 28–July 1, 1969, at the Stonewall Inn, a gay club in Greenwich Village in New York City) or other LGBTQ+ activist events.

- Sapiosexual: Someone who is attracted to people based on their intelligence.

Terms to Avoid

When you encounter someone for the first time, use the name they've indicated they want to be called and the pronouns they've asked to be used. When in doubt, the singular use of the pronoun, they, is usually considered gender-neutral and respectful. Try not to place quotations around someone's name or pronouns—even in your mind!

Many of the terms listed below are considered slurs. Slurs can be reclaimed, as mentioned above, so it's possible that people do use them to refer to themselves. However, unless a person has told you it's OK to use the following in describing them, it's safest to avoid these terms altogether.

- Homosexual: This is an outdated and more medicalized term to describe gay and lesbian people.
- Sexual preference: Sexual orientation is not a preference.
- Preferred pronouns: Pronouns aren't preferred or optional. They're required in respectful relationships.

- Fag, dyke, homo: Slurs for gay men, lesbians, and both, respectively.
- Sodomite, deviant, diseased, perverted

Note: "-Phobia/-phobic" (fear) is the traditional suffix for some terms explored in this section. However, that suffix is also ableist—meaning, discriminatory against people who have legitimate phobias. Bigotry is not a mental health issue and should not be treated as such—doing so is harmful to those with mental health diseases. The suffix -misia/-misic (-misia is pronounced miz-eeya), from the Greek word for hate or hatred, is used in place of -phobia here to be less harmful and more linguistically precise. (Simmons Library, 2018)

- Bimisia: Bigotry and discrimination against bisexual people. This is usually seen in how people label relationships of bisexual people (e.g., a bisexual woman dating another woman is often called a lesbian, but if she's dating a man she's called straight).
- Closeted: Someone who has not disclosed their sexual orientation to others; someone who isn't "out" about their sexual orientation (or gender).
- Coming out: The process someone takes when they share their sexual orientation with others, either publicly or privately. This isn't an all-or-nothing process—for example, someone can "come out" to friends but stay closeted to their parents.
- Heteronormativity: The societal assumption that every relationship will be heterosexual. This message is often sent to us in media we

experience, such as ads or television shows featuring a large majority of heterosexual couples. This can also be called heterosexism.

- Homomisia: Bigotry and discrimination against gay men and lesbians.
- Outing: Sharing someone's sexual orientation without their permission, particularly when they're closeted.
- Questioning: Someone who is unsure of or exploring their sexual orientation.

Appendix C: Gender Identity

By Kirsten Schultz, MS

It's only in recent years that more research has led to a better understanding of gender. Gender identity is simply someone's gender, which is based on how they feel, and not on physical characteristics. How they share their gender with the outside world, through how they dress and act, contributes to their gender expression. These terms are important to understanding gender overall:

- AFAB: Assigned female at birth.
- AMAB: Assigned male at birth.
- Femme: This can be a shorthand for feminine. Femmes usually have a more feminine gender expression. It can also denote a non-binary person who presents more feminine as well as a cisgender woman who embraces her femininity.
- Masc: This can be a shorthand for masculine or someone who has a more masculine gender expression. It can denote a non-binary person who presents more masculine as well as a cisgender man who embraces their masculinity.

Gender Terms

- Agender or gender neutrois: Does not have a gender.
- Androgynous: Appearing gender neutral.
- Aporagender: A strong gender identity that is neither male nor female.

- Bigender: Encompassing male and female gender identities. Ambigender is a similar term.
- Butch: A more masculine gender expression from someone who is AFAB.
- Cisgender: Someone who identifies as the gender they were assigned at birth.
- Demigender: Non-binary but feeling that one is partly a certain gender.
    o Demiboy: Feeling partially like a boy.
    o Demigirl: Feeling partially like a girl.
- Gender fluid: Someone who does not have a fixed gender, but feels as though their gender is a range.
- Gender neutral: Someone who doesn't feel as though they're one gender or another. This can be a term applied to items as well, such as gender-neutral bathrooms, etc.
- Gender non-conforming (GNC): Someone who doesn't conform to societal gender ideas or the gender binary.
- Genderqueer: Someone who is GNC and defies gender norms by identifying as no gender, bigender, or some combination or a variety of genders.
- Intersex: Someone who was born with a combination of male and female anatomy and/or chromosomes.
    o Intergender: An intersex-specific gender identity denoting a combination of masc/femme gender identities; similar to genderqueer or

androgynous.

- o (Antonym) Dyadic: Someone who is not intersex.
- Metrosexual: A cisgender man who pays more attention to his appearance. This term peaked in the early 2000s and is now rarely used due to a growing understanding of various genders and gender roles.
- Non-binary: Someone who does not fit into the gender binary.
- Pangender: Being more than one gender or being all genders.
- Transgender: Someone who was assigned a certain gender at birth but is not that gender.
  - o Transitioning: The process of matching one's body to one's gender. The gender affirming process is often a long and difficult one. It is important to keep in mind that not everyone can or wants to undergo any or all of these steps:
    - Gender affirming hormone treatment (HRT): Hormones are started to help the development of desired gender traits. This can include estrogen, antiandrogens, progesterone, testosterone, androgens, antiestrogens, and more. Depending on delivery method and needs, these may be taken daily. Close attention should be paid to patients with contraindicated conditions including liver or kidney

disease and migraines.

- Surgeries
  - Top surgery: Surgery to alter a person's chest. Depending on the person's gender, this would be either breast augmentation or bilateral mastectomy and chest reconstruction.
  - Bottom surgery: There are a variety of surgeries that may be needed for bottom surgery. Patients may need a hysterectomy, bilateral salpingo-oophorectomy, vaginectomy, penectomy, and/or orchiectomy. A vaginoplasty creates a vagina and vulva from the patient's penis and surrounding material. Surgeries that aid in the creation of a penis can include scrotoplasty, metoidioplasty, and phalloplasty.
  - Additional surgery: Surgery can be had to assist with facial feminization, vocal feminization, tracheal shave, and buttock augmentation.
- Trans man: Someone who was assigned female at birth and is more masc. This does not require any HRT or surgery. Additional terms include trans masc or FTM (female-to-male).
- Trans woman: Someone who was assigned male at birth and is more femme. This does not require any HRT or surgery. Additional terms include trans femme or MTF (male-to-female).
- Gender bender: Someone who constantly

defies societal rules of gender identity and/or expression. They may work to defy these things intentionally or do so unintentionally.

- Fooling/pretending: This is often used when someone feels as though they've been fooled by someone of another gender (generally a transgender person). There are those whose transmisia runs deep enough that they believe trans people try to fool or trick them into relationships. No person pretends to be another gender for those reasons.

Trans-related Terms to Avoid

- Transgendered: Transgender is a noun, not a verb. The correct term would be someone who is transgender.
- Transgenders: This removes someone's humanity. The correct term here would be transgender (or trans) people.
- A transgender: This removes someone's humanity. Use a transgender (or trans) person.
- Tranny/trannie: A shortened form of transgender, generally used as a slur.
- Transsexual: This is an outdated term for trans people.
- Transvestite: An outdated term for cross-dresser.
- Sex change or pre-op/post-op: These phrases place the focus on the state of a person's genitals, not their gender.
- She-male, he-she, it: These phrases remove a

person's humanity.
- Passing: Someone whose gender expression matches assumptions about what people of their gender look like. This is usually used to refer to someone who is transgender but can "pass" as cisgender. Because of the harm of a focus on passing, this is not a favored term in non-cisgender circles.

Other Terms
- Cishet: Cisgender and heterosexual.
- Cisheterosexism: The societal favoring of cisgender and heterosexual people.
- Cissexism: The societal favoring of cisgender people.
- Drag: People of one gender who dress up as another gender for performances.
- Genderism: A belief in the gender binary or that there are only two genders.
- Mx (mix): A gender-neutral replacement for Miss/Ms., Mister/Mr., or Misses/Mrs.
- Stealth: Someone who is trans but not "out" about their gender.
- Transmisia: Bigotry or discrimination against transgender people.

Commonly Used Pronouns

People, regardless of gender, may prefer to be addressed using a wide variety of pronouns. Below is a list of commonly used pronouns with pronunciation in parentheses and italics. Please note that this list is not exhaustive.

- She/her
- He/him
- They/them
- Ze/zir *(zee/zere)* or ze/hir *(zee/here)*
- Ey/em *(eh/'em)* or ey/eir *(eh/'ers)*
- Ve/vir *(vee/veer)*
- Xe/xem *(zee/zem)* or xe/xim *(zee/zim)* or xe/hir *(zee/here)* or xe/xym *(zee/zim)*

Many more pronouns exist, and there are excellent academic sources on them for anyone wishing to learn more (Lesbian, Gay, Bisexual, Transgender Resource Center, 2018). If you make a mistake regarding someone's pronouns or gender, don't panic. Those of us who aren't cisgender or who use different pronouns completely understand. The best way to react is to apologize and correct yourself, and then move on.

Appendix D: Gender and Culture

By Kirsten Schultz, MS

Historically, Westernized civilization has embraced a *gender binary*—the idea that someone is either a woman or a man based on their genitals or sex. Most people are assigned male or female at birth. Along with this binary is an assumption of certain gender roles that generally see women as homemakers and caretakers while men work outside the home. However, that's not the way that many cultures have seen, experienced, or expressed gender. Here are just a few culturally specific gender terms:

- Fa'afafine (Samoa and Polynesia): Fa'afafine (fa-ahfa-een) are assigned male at birth (AMAB) and embody both feminine and masculine traits. They engage in traditionally feminine tasks during childhood and adulthood. The majority of fa'afafine are accepted throughout society as a third gender.
- Hijra (India and South Asia): While hijra (hidj-ra) can refer to people who are eunuchs and intersex, it is most commonly used toward transgender people who were assigned male at birth (AMAB). Hijras take on more feminine features, clothing, and tasks as they grow up. With the help of a guide, they may undergo surgery to complete their transitioning process. Hijra is a recognized third gender across India, Bangladesh, Nepal, and Pakistan.
- Khanith (Oman and the Middle East): Khanith (kaan-ith) refers to AMAB individuals who fill

feminine roles in relationships with other men as well as in their social lives. The khanith are still treated as men in society and called by their birth name. It's also interesting to note that people may give up the khanith lifestyle for heterosexual marriage and a family.

- Two Spirit (Indigenous North America): While there are many gender terms used across North America, the most well-known is Two Spirit. This term can apply to a range of people, from transgender and intersex individuals to those who express their gender identities in unique ways. Two Spirit people have always been, and continue to be, respected members of their communities.

- Muxe (Mexico): Muxe (moo-shay) people are AMAB while engaging in traditionally feminine tasks, usually from a young age. These individuals can express their gender either by wearing feminine clothing or combining male clothing with makeup. As with many transgender individuals, muxes may take hormones and strive to transition—or not. Each person makes decisions that fit them regarding expression and transition.

There are many more examples, from Hawaii to Madagascar, and as far back as to the time of the Incas (Bader, 2014; Diavolo, 2017). Many of these communities did not see varying genders as negative until colonization from Western civilizations.

References

About Masters & Johnson.
https://kinseyinstitute.org/collections/archival/mast
ers-and-johnson.php. Accessed March 17, 2019.

About Recreational Therapy.
https://www.nctrc.org/about-ncrtc/about-
recreational-therapy/. Accessed August 5, 2020.

Act Against AIDS.
https://www.cdc.gov/actagainstaids/campaigns/start
talking/. Accessed May 30, 2019.

Alammyan A. What Does it Feel Like to Go From
Physically Unattractive to Attractive?
https://www.quora.com/What-does-it-feel-like-to-
go-from-physically-unattractive-to-attractive-What-
kind-of-reactions-did-you-get-from-strangers-before-
and-after-How-did-it-change-you-Do-you-now-take-
advantage-of-your-looks. Accessed December 12,
2018.

Alternatives to intercourse.
https://smartsexresource.com/topics/alternatives-to-
intercourse. Accessed December 17, 2019.

Alterowitz R, Alterowitz B. Impotence After Prostate
Cancer.
https://www.hisprostatecancer.com/impotence.html.
Accessed October 3, 2019.

Anderson JB. STID? [Sexually transmissible infectious
disease]: The case for a new term.
www.ashasexualhealth.org/stid-the-case-for-a-new-
term/. Accessed December 17, 2019.

References

Anti-oppression: What Does "Misia" Mean?
https://simmons.libguides.com/anti-oppression#s-lib-ctab-10174165-1. Accessed February 1, 2018.

Bader L. Third Genders: New Concept? Or Old?
https://sites.psu.edu/evolutionofhumansexuality/2014/02/19/third-genders-new-concept-or-old/.
Accessed October 3, 2019.

Bagemihl B. Biological exuberance: animal homosexuality and natural diversity. New York, NY: St. Martin's Press; 1999.

Basson R. The Female Sexual Response: A Different Model. *The Journal of Sex & Marital Therapy.* 2000; 26(1):51-65. Abstract.

Bates L. The Trouble With Sex Robots.
https://www.nytimes.com/2017/07/17/opinion/sex-robots-consent.html. Accessed April 2, 2019.

Baum N. Forget the PC Police and Telemedicine: Give Your Patient a Hug.
https://www.kevinmd.com/blog/2018/01/forget-pc-police-telemedicine-give-patient-hug.html. Accessed December 2, 2019.

Berman L. *The Sex Ed Handbook: A Comprehensive Guide for Parents.*
http://media.oprah.com/lberman/talking-to-kids-about-sex-handbook.pdf. Accessed June 22, 2020.

Beyond Intercourse.
https://www.breastcancer.org/tips/intimacy/beyond. Accessed December 3, 2019.

Bitzer J, Giacomo P, Tschudin S, et al. Sexual Counseling for Women in the Context of Physical Diseases: A Teaching Model for Physicians. *The Journal of Sexual Medicine.* 2007; 4, 29-37.

Blodgett, G. *Understanding Patients' Sexual Problems: A Reference Handbook for Healthcare Professionals.* New York, NY: Aviva Publishing; 2015.

Braford J, McKenzie N. Menopause, Manopause, and Redefining Sexuality. Lecture presented at: 14th Annual Art & Science of Aging Conference – Revisiting Relationships: Intimate, Intergenerational, and More; February 22, 2019; Grand Rapids, Mich.

Brambilla C. From Virtual Reality Porn To Sex Robots— How Adult Entertainment Is Rapidly Changing. https://www.newsweek.com/virtual-reality-porn-sex-robots-how-adult-entertainment-rapidly-changing-1257375. Accessed March 25, 2019.

Castleman M. Men's Secret Sex Problem. https://www.aarp.org/relationships/love-sex/info-11-2010/men_sex_problem_cannot_climax.html. Accessed October 10, 2019.

Cavanaugh S. Four Steps to Resuming a Healthy Sex Life After Cancer. https://www.cancercenter.com/community/blog/2015/09/four-steps-to-resuming-a-healthy-sex-life-after-cancer. Accessed October 3, 2019.

Changes in Your Sex Life. https://www.breastcancer.org/tips/intimacy/changes. Accessed October 3, 2019.

Chapman G. *The Five Love Languages: How to Express Heartfelt Commitment to Your Mate.* Chicago, Ill: Northfield Publishing; 2014.

Clayton A, Ramamurthy S. The Impact of Physical Illness on Sexual Dysfunction. *Advances in Psychosomatic Medicine.* 2008; 29: 70-88. Abstract.

Cohen D, Gonzalez J. The Role of Pelvic Floor Muscles in Male Sexual Dysfunction and Pelvic Pain. *Sexual Medicine Reviews*. 2016; Vol. 4, Issue 1;53-62.

Daleboudt GMN, Broadbent E, McQueen F, and Kaptein K. The Impact of Illness Perceptions on Sexual Functioning in Patients with Systemic Lupus Erythematosus. *The Journal of Psychosomatic Research*. 2013; 74; 260-264.

Dare to Care: Guide to Partner Communication. Navy and Marine Corp Public Health Center. https://www.med.navy.mil/sites/nmcphc/Document s/health-promotion-wellness/wounded-ill-and-injured/WII-Toolbox/Relationships-and-Intimacy/WII_RelAndInt_PartnerGuide.pdf. Accessed April 13, 2020.

Davidson E. The Sneaky Perks of Dating Someone with Rheumatoid Arthritis. https://creakyjoints.org/sex-and-intimacy/benefits-dating-someone-with-arthritis/. Accessed February 20, 2020.

Dee J. Thirteen Ways to Be More Present During Sex. https://www.uncoveringintimacy.com/13-ways-present-sex/. Accessed October 3, 2019.

Defining pornography. https://www.merriamwebster.com/dictionary/porno graphy. Accessed May 27, 2020.

Defining sexual health. https://www.who.int/reproductivehealth/topics/sex ual_health/sh_definitions/en/. Accessed April 17, 2019.

Diavolo L. Gender Variance Around the World Over Time. https://www.teenvogue.com/story/gender-variance-around-the-world. Accessed October 3,

2019.

Digital Get Down.
https://www.goodvibes.com/s/good-vibes-buzz/sex-tips-tricks/digital-get-down. Accessed July 16, 2020.

Duke K. *Kissability: People With Disabilities Talk About Sex, Love, and Relationships*. Amherst, Mass: Levellers Press; 2014.

Edwards KA, Alschuler KA, Ehde DM, Battalio SL, Jensen MP. Changes in resilience predict function in adults with physical disabilities: A longitudinal study. *Archives of Physical Medicine and Rehabilitation*. 2017; Vol. 98, Issue 2.

Evan E, Kaufman M, Cook A, Zeltzer L. Sexual health and self-esteem in adolescents and young adults with cancer. *Cancer*. 2006; Vol. 107, Issue S7.

Evans S. The Lesser Known Erogenous Zones—And How To Find Them. https://www.independent.co.uk/life-style/love-sex/the-lesser-known-erogenous-zones-and-how-to-find-them-10419267.html#comments. Accessed October 3, 2019.

Evans S. Sex Toy Tips.
https://www.jodivine.com/articles/sex-toy-tips/sex-aids. Accessed July 17, 2020.

Flynn KE, Lin L, Bruner DW, et al. Sexual satisfaction and the importance of sexual health to quality of life throughout the life course of US adults. *The Journal of Sexual Medicine*. 2016. November 13(11): 1642-1650.

Gender Pronouns.
https://uwm.edu/lgbtrc/support/gender-pronouns/. Accessed October 3, 2019.

Gordon LH. Intimacy: The Art of Relationships. *Psychology Today*.

https://www.psychologytoday.com/articles/196912/i
ntimacy-the-art-relationships. Accessed October 3,
2019.

Gould WR. What is maintenance sex? It may help strengthen
your marriage. https://www.nbcnews.com/better/pop-
culture/what-maintenance-sex-it-may-help-strengthen-
your-marriage-ncna956216. Accessed June 29, 2020.

Fixter A. The taboos around disability and sex put limits
on everyone, disabled or not.
https://www.theguardian.com/commentisfree/2019/
mar/18/disabled-people-sexuality-dating-society-
taboo-marginalise. Accessed June 25, 2020.

Healey E, Haywood K, Jordan K, et al. Ankylosing
spondylitis and its impact on sexual relationships.
Rheumatology. 2009; 48(17);1378-1381.

Hensel DJ, Nance J, Fortenberry JD. The Association
Between Sexual Health and Physical, Mental, and
Social Health in Adolescent Women. *The Journal of
Adolescent Health.* 2016; October;59(4):416-21.

HIV Among People Aged 50 and Older. Centers for
Disease Control and Prevention.
https://www.cdc.gov/hiv/group/age/olderamericans
/index.html. Accessed October 3, 2019.

Hutcherson H. After Hysterectomy, A New Approach to
Sex and Orgasm.
https://womensvoicesforchange.org/after-
hysterectomy-a-new-approach-to-sex-and-
orgasm.htm. Accessed October 3, 2019.

I don't feel attractive enough to be with my partner.
https://www.relate.org.uk/relationship-help/help-
relationships/mental-health/i-dont-feel-attractive-
enough-be-my-partner. Accessed December 5, 2018.

Is Sex In Later Years Good for Your Health?
http://msutoday.msu.edu/news/2016/is-sex-in-later-
years-good-for-your-health/?utm_campaign=media-
pitch&utm_medium=email. Accessed February 1,
2018.

Jameson M. Seniors' sex lives are up—and so are STD
cases around the country.
http://articles.orlandosentinel.com/2011-05-
16/health/os-seniors-stds-national-20110516_1_std-
cases-syphilis-and-chlamydia-older-adults/. Accessed
February 1, 2018.

Jedel S, Hood MH, Keshavarzian A. Getting Personal: A
Review of Sexual Functioning, Body Image, and Their
Impact on Quality of Life in IBD Patients.
Inflammatory Bowel Diseases. 2015; April;21(4):923-
938.

Kaufman M, Silverberg C, Odette F. *The Ultimate Guide
to Sex and Disability: For All of Us Who Live with
Disabilities, Chronic Pain, and Illness.* 2nd ed. Jersey
City, NJ: Cleis Press; 2007.

Kessler D. https://grief.com/the-five-stages-of-grief/.
Accessed December 5, 2019.

Klein A. *Learning to Laugh When You Feel Like Crying:
Embracing Life After Loss.* Norwood, NJ: Goodman
Beck Publishing; 2011.

Klein MJ. Sexuality and Disability.
https://emedicine.medscape.com/article/319119-
overview. Accessed December 5, 2019.

Krischer H. 7 Awesome Erogenous Zones.
https://www.webmd.com/sex-
relationships/features/7-awesome-erogenous-
zones#2. Accessed December 11, 2018.

Lack of Sexual Desire and/or Arousal.
https://sexualadviceassociation.co.uk/lack-sexual-desire-andor-arousal/. Accessed March 15, 2018.

Lavernia CJ, Villa JM. High Rates of Interest in Sex in Patients with Hip Arthritis. *Clinical Orthopedics and Related Research.* 2016;474:293-299.

Learn How to Choose Your First Sex Toy.
https://www.comeasyouare.com/blogs/sex-information/how-to-choose-your-first-sex-toy?_pos=1&_sid=b3c465228&_ss=r. Accessed July 17, 2020.

Leavitt CE, Lefkowitz ES, Waterman EA. The Role of Sexual Mindfulness in Sexual Wellbeing, Relational Wellbeing, and Self-esteem. *The Journal of Sex and Marital Therapy.* 2019; 45(6): 497–509.

Levis B, Burri A, Hudson M, Baron M, et al. Sexual Activity and Impairment in Women With Systemic Sclerosis Compared to Women From a General Population Sample. *PLOS ONE.* 2012. December; Vol. 7, Issue 12.

Lieberman H. In Defense of Sex Robots.
https://qz.com/1215360/in-defense-of-sex-robots/. Accessed March 22, 2019.

Liu H, Waite LJ, Shen S, Wang DH. Is Sex Good for Your Health? A National Study on Partnered Sexuality and Cardiovascular Risk Among Older Men and Women. *Journal of Health and Social Behavior.* 2016. 57(3): 276-296.

Lunelli RP, Rabello ER, Stein R, Goldmeier S, et al. Sexual Activity after MI: Taboo or Lack of Knowledge? *Arquivos brasileiros de cardiologia.* 2008; 90(3): 156-159.

MacHattie E, Naphtali K, Elliott S. *PleasurABLE: A Sexual Device Manual for Persons with Disabilities.* Vancouver, British Columbia, Canada; self-published; 2009.

McGuire J. Experts Tell Us 13 Ways to Have the Best Sex Ever.https://www.esquire.com/lifestyle/sex/g622/better-sex/. Accessed December 17, 2018.

Mosack V, Steinke E. Trends in Sexual Concerns After MI. *Journal of Cardiovascular Nursing.* 2009; 24(2), 162-170.

Mosher DL. Three Dimensions of Depth of Involvement in Human Sexual Response. *The Journal of Sex Research.* 1980; Vol. 16, Issue 1.

OXO: Our Philosophy. https://www.oxo.com/aboutus. Accessed August 4, 2020.

Pakpour AH, Nikoobakht M, Campbell P. Association of Pain and Depression in Those With Chronic Back Pain: The Mediation Effect of Patient Sexual Functioning. *Clinical Journal of Pain.* 2015; Volume 31, Number 1; 44-51.

Park A. "Sexual Healing" (2004). *Time Magazine* 163(3), 76-77.

Pelon S, Huang L. Sexual Health Promotion in Long Term Care. Lecture presented at: 14th Annual Art & Science of Aging Conference – Revisiting Relationships: Intimate, Intergenerational, and More. February 22, 2019; Grand Rapids, Mich.

Pfaus JG, Quintana GR, Cionnaith CM, Parada M. The Whole Versus the Sum of Some of the Parts: Toward Resolving the Apparent Controversy of Clitoral Versus Vaginal Orgasms. *Socioaffective Neuroscience*

& *Psychology*. 2016; 6: 10.3402.

Pillai-Friedman S. How to Talk to Your Doctor About Sexuality Issues. https://community.breastcancer.org/blog/how-to-talk-to-your-doctor-about-sexuality-issues. Accessed September 28, 2019.

Pope NK, Voges KE, Kuhn KL, Bloxsome EL. Pornography and Erotica: Definitions and Prevalence. Proceedings of the 2007 International Nonprofit and Social Marketing Conference: Social Entrepreneurship, Social Change and Sustainability, Griffith University, Brisbane, Australia.

Quinn-Nilas C, Benson L, Milhausen RR, et al. The Relationship Between Body Image and Domains of Sexual Functioning Among Heterosexual, Emerging Adult Women. *The Journal of Sexual Medicine*. 2016; September;4(3):182-9.

Robinson KM. 10 Surprising Health Benefits of Sex. https://www.webmd.com/sex-relationships/guide/sex-and-health#1. Accessed October 10, 2019.

Russell B. (1929). Marriage and Morals. Retrieved from: https://en.wikiquote.org/wiki/Marriage_and_Morals

Sex and Disability: The Facts. https://www.aruma.com.au/about-us/blog/sex-and-disability-the-facts. Accessed December 3, 2019.

Sex-Drive Killers. https://www.webmd.com/sexual-conditions/ss/slideshow-sex-drive-killers. Accessed January 20, 2019.

Sexual Health Coloring Book. Durham, North Carolina: American Sexual Health Association; 2019.

Sexuality and Relationships, in "A Strategy for Equality." http://nda.ie/Disability-overview/Key-Policy-Documents/Report-of-the-Commission-on-the-Status-of-People-with-Disabilities/A-Strategy-for-Equality/A-Strategy-for-Equality-Report-of-the-Commission-on-the-Status-of-People-with-Disabilities/Sexuality-and-relationships. Accessed February 13, 2020.

Shifren JL, Hanfling S, eds. *Sexuality in Midlife and Beyond*. Boston, Mass: Harvard Health Publications; 2015.

Siegel AL. Pelvic Floor Muscle Training in Males: Practical Applications. *Urology*. 2014; 84;1; 1-7.

Silva CMC, Santos IMM, Vargens OMC. Woman experiencing gynecologic surgery: coping with the changes imposed by surgery. *Revista Latino-Americana de Enfermagem*, 2016;24.

Slattery J. *No More Headaches: Enjoying Sex & Intimacy in Marriage*. Carol Stream, Ill: Tyndale House Publishers; 2009.

Taylor PC, Moore A, Vasilescu R, et al. A structured literature review of the burden of illness and unmet needs in patients with rheumatoid arthritis: a current perspective. *Rheumatology International*. 2016; 36:685–695.

Thomson H. Women don't need to 'switch off' to climax, orgasm study shows. https://www.newscientist.com/article/2150180-women-dont-need-to-switch-off-to-climax-orgasm-study-shows/ Accessed December 4, 2019.

Turning a wheelchair into a love seat.
https://www.metrotimes.com/detroit/turning-a-wheelchair-into-a-love-seat/Content?oid=2183333.
Accessed March 25, 2019.

Understanding Sexual Health.
http://ashasexualhealth.org/sexual-health/. Accessed July 26, 2019.

University of Washington (2016). How to Bounce Back [Factsheet]. Aging Well with a Physical Disability Factsheet Series. Healthy Aging & Physical Disability Rehabilitation Research & Training Center.
http://agerrtc.washington.edu/info/factsheets/resilience. Accessed April 12, 2020. (The Healthy Aging RRTC officially closed in September 2018. The information posted online remains as a historical record of the projects, research, and members of the RRTC.)

Wittmann D, Carolan M, Given B, et al. What Couples Say about Their Recovery of Sexual Intimacy after Prostatectomy: Toward the Development of a Conceptual Model of Couples' Sexual Recovery after Surgery for Prostate Cancer. *Journal of Sexual Medicine.* 2015; February: 12(2): 494-504.
  You and Your Partner.
http://www.breastcancer.org/tips/intimacy/partner. Accessed October 3, 2019.

Zahlis EH, Lewis FM. Coming to Grips with Breast Cancer: The Spouse's Experience with His Wife's First Six Months. *Journal of Psychosocial Oncology.* 2010; 28(1): 79–97.

Recommended Reading

Brisben, Patty. *Pure Romance Between the Sheets: Find Your Best Sexual Self and Enhance Your Intimate Relationship.* Atria Books; Reprint edition; 2015.

Brotto, Lori. *Better Sex Through Mindfulness: How Women Can Cultivate Desire.* Simon & Schuster; 2015.

Chapman, Gary. *The Five Love Languages: How to Express Heartfelt Commitment to Your Mate.* Northfield Publishing; 2014.

Cox, Tracey. *Supersex for Life: The Great Sex Guide for Long-Term Lovers.* DK ADULT; 2010.

Cox, Tracey. *Great Sex Starts at 50: How to Age-Proof Your Libido.* Murdoch Books; 2020.

Duke, Katherine. *Kissability: People with Disabilities Talk About Sex, Love, and Relationships.* Levellers Press; 2014.

Foley, Sallie; Kope, Sally; Sugrue, Dennis. *Sex Matters for Women: A Complete Guide to Taking Care of Your Sexual Self.* Guilford Press; Second edition; 2011.

Gungor, Mark. *Laugh Your Way to a Better Marriage.* Atria Books; Reprint edition, 2009.

Joannides, Paul. *Guide To Getting It On: Unzipped.* Goofy Foot Press; Ninth edition; 2017.

Kaufman, Miriam; Silverberg, Cory; Odette, Fran. *The Ultimate Guide to Sex and Disability: For All of Us Who Live with Disabilities, Chronic Pain, and Illness.* Cleis Press; Second edition; 2007.

Lipton, Benjamin. *Gay Men Living with Chronic Illnesses and Disabilities: From Crisis to Crossroads.* Routledge; 2004.

Nagoski, Emily. *Come as You Are: The Surprising New Science that Will Transform Your Sex Life.* Greystone Books; 2018.

Napthtali, Kate; MacHattie, Edith; Elliott, Stacy. *PleasurABLE Sexual Device Manual for Persons with Disabilities.* Self-published; 2009.

Price, Joan. *Naked at Our Age: Talking Out Loud About Senior Sex.* Seal Press; 2011.

Resources

Basic Sexual Education

Answer: Sex Ed Honestly: Resources for Professionals –
http://answer.rutgers.edu/page/resources
American Association of Sex Educators, Counselors, and
Therapists - www.aasect.org
The American Board of Sexology –
http://theamericanboardofsexology.com
CreakyJoints.org - https://creakyjoints.org/?s=sex
Dr. Tina Schermer Sellers -
www.tinaschermersellers.com
Gender Identity & Pronoun Use: A Guide For
Pediatric Health Care Professionals –
https://notes.childrenshospital.org/clinicians-guide-
gender-identity-pronoun-use/
The Gender Unicorn - www.transstudent.org/gender
Gingerbread Person -
http://itspronouncedmetrosexual.com/2015/03/the-
genderbread-person-v3/
Great Sex Guidance - https://greatsexguidance.com/
International Society of the Study of Women's Sexual
Health - www.isswsh.org
National Association of Nurse Practitioners in Women's
Health - www.npwh.org
The North American Menopause Society –
www.menopause.org
National Coalition for Sexual Freedom –
https://ncsfreedom.org
National LGBT Health Education Center: Learning

Modules -
www.lgbthealtheducation.org/resources/type/learnin
g-module/
SafeSexResource - https://smartsexresource.com/
Scarleteen: Sex Education for the Real World –
www.scarleteen.com/
Sexual Advice Association –
https://sexualadviceassociation.co.uk
Sexual Health: An Adolescent Provider Toolkit –
https://partnerships.ucsf.edu/sites/partnerships.ucsf
.edu/files/images/SexualHealthToolkit2010BW.pdf
The Sexuality Information and Education Council of the
U.S. - https://siecus.org
The Society of Sex Therapy and Research –
www.sstarnet.org
Start Talking Stop HIV –
www.cdc.gov/actagainstaids/campaigns/starttalking
/index.html
UW-Milwaukee: Gender Pronouns –
http://uwm.edu/lgbtrc/support/gender-pronouns/

Disability

Ability Online for youth with disabilities, parents and
professionals -www.abilityonline.org
Aruma - www.hwns.com.au
Association of University Centers on Disabilities –
www.aucd.org/template/index.cfm
Come As You Are Co-operative -
www.comeasyouare.com
Dare to CARE –
www.med.navy.mil/sites/nmcphc/Documents/health

-promotion-wellness/wounded-ill-and-injured/WII-Toolbox/Relationships-and-Intimacy/WII_RelAndInt_PartnerGuide.pdf

Four Things Healthcare Providers Need to Know About Sexuality and Disability - http://readysexyable.com/ready/2016/04/20/to-healthcare-providers-what-wed-like-you-to-know-about-sexuality-and-disability/

How Chronic Illness Can Affect Sexual Function – www.aasect.org/how-chronic-illness-can-affect-sexual-function

How Crohn's Affects Your Sexuality and Intimacy www.crohnsandme.com/living-with-crohns-disease/crohns-disease-and-sex.aspx

Real RA: It's Not Just About the Jar – http://theseatedview.blogspot.com/2012/01/real-ra-its-not-just-about-jar.html?spref=tw

Sex with Arthritis: Everyday Health – www.everydayhealth.com/specialists/arthritis/kitridou/qa/sex-with-arthritis.aspx

Sex and Disability: Come As You Are Cooperative – www.comeasyouare.com/sex-information/sex-and-disability/

Sex and Disability: The Center for Sexual Health and Pleasure (CSPH) - www.thecsph.org/the-csph-resources/web-resources/sex-and/sex-and-disability/

Sex and Disability Speakers   - www.chronicsex.org/sex-disability-speakers/

Sexuality Education for Youth with Disability or Chronic Illness. www.med.umich.edu/yourchild/topics/disabsex.htm

Sexual Positioning Devices –

http://atwiki.assistivetech.net/index.php/Sexual_Pos
itioning_Devices
Study Shows One-Third Of Rheumatoid Arthritis Patients
Experience Sexual Dysfunction -
https://rheumatoidarthritis.net/living/study-shows-
one-third-of-patients-experience-sexual-dysfunction/

LGBT+ Health

10 Tips for Working with Transgender Patients: An
Information and Resource Publication for Healthcare
Providers - http://transgenderlawcenter.org/wp-
content/uploads/2011/12/01.28.2016-tips-
healthcare.pdf
Affirmative Care for Transgender and Gender Non-
Conforming People: Best Practices for Front-line
Health Care Staff - www.lgbthealtheducation.org/wp-
content/uploads/13-
017_TransBestPracticesforFrontlineStaff_v6_02-19-
13_FINAL.pdf
A Resource Roundup for Aspiring Allies to Transgender,
Gender-Variant, Intersex, & Nonbinary Folks -
https://medium.com/athena-talks/because-not-
everybody-can-just-google-it-a-resource-round-up-
for-self-education-regarding-43eb57979171
Asking Patients Questions about Sexual Orientation and
Gender Identity in Clinical Settings: A Study in Four
Health Centers - http://thefenwayinstitute.org/wp-
content/uploads/COM228_SOGI_CHARN_WhitePape
r.pdf
Best Practices for Asking Questions to Identify
Transgender and Other Gender Minority

Respondents on Population-Based Surveys - https://williamsinstitute.law.ucla.edu/wp-content/uploads/geniuss-report-sep-2014.pdf

Collecting Sexual Orientation and Gender Identity Data in Electronic Health Records: Workshop Summary - www.ncbi.nlm.nih.gov/books/NBK154082/

Lesbian, Gay, Bisexual, and Transgender-Related Content in Undergraduate Medical Education – https://jamanetwork.com/journals/jama/fullarticle/1104294

Non-Binary Gender Identities Factsheet from the Society for the Psychological Study of Lesbian, Gay, Bisexual, and Transgender Issues - www.apadivisions.org/division-44/resources/advocacy/non-binary-facts.pdf

Patterns and Predictors of Disclosure of Sexual Orientation to Healthcare Providers among Lesbians, Gay Men, and Bisexuals - https://williamsinstitute.law.ucla.edu/research/health-and-hiv-aids/durso-meyer-srsp-dec-2012/

Stanford University Study: Discrimination fears remain for LGBT medical students – https://med.stanford.edu/news/all-news/2015/02/many-lgbt-medical-students-choose-to-stay-in-the-closet.html

Ten Things Bisexuals Should Discuss with Their Healthcare Provider - http://glma.org/index.cfm?fuseaction=Page.ViewPage&PageID=1026

Ten Things Gay Men Should Discuss with Their Healthcare Provider - http://glma.org/index.cfm?fuseaction=Page.viewPag

e&pageID=690

Ten Things Transgender Persons Should Discuss with Their Healthcare Care Provider - www.glma.org/index.cfm?fuseaction=Page.viewPage &pageID=692

Top 10 Things Lesbians Should Discuss with Their Healthcare Provider - www.glma.org/index.cfm?fuseaction=Page.viewPage &pageID=691

Transgender Health: Patients & Providers Series – https://genderqueer.me/transgender-patients-providers/

Yes, Your Doctor Really Needs to Ask About Your Sexual Orientation & Gender Identity - www.slate.com/blogs/outward/2016/02/29/why_do ctors_need_to_ask_patients_about_sexuality_and_ge nder_identity.html

LBGTQ+ Organizations

Arkansas Transgender Equality Coalition

Equitas Health Institute for LGBTQ Health Equity – http://equitashealthinstitute.com/

Los Angeles LGBT Center - https://lalgbtcenter.org/

Mazzoni Center: LGBT Health and Well-Being – www.mazzonicenter.org/

National Center for Lesbian Rights - www.nclrights.org/

National Coalition for Sexual Freedom – https://ncsfreedom.org/

National LGBT Cancer Network – https://cancer-network.org/

National LGBT Health Education Center –

www.lgbthealtheducation.org/
Pride Center of Vermont - www.pridecentervt.org/
The Montrose Center - www.montrosecenter.org/hub/
The SF LGBT Center - www.sfcenter.org/
TransAdvocate - http://transadvocate.com/
Whitman-Walker Health - www.whitman-walker.org/
World Professional Association for Transgender Health
    www.wpath.org/
Zami Nobla: National Organization of Black Lesbians on
    Aging - https://zaminobla.org/

Non-Monogamy and Polyamory

Polyamory-Friendly Professionals Directory –
    http://polyfriendly.org/list.php?category=Medical%2
    oProfessionals
What Healthcare Professionals Need to Know About Poly
    and Kink - http://polyweekly.com/what-healthcare-
    professionals-need-to-know-about-poly-and-kink/
Why Doctors Need to Pay More Attention to Their Kinky
    Patients -https://qz.com/342268/why-doctors-need-
    to-pay-more-attention-to-their-kinky-patients/

People, Organizations, and Centers

Andrew Gurza is a queer Canadian man living with
    cerebral palsy who focuses on shedding light on the
    intersections of disability, queerness, and sexuality –
    www.andrewgurza.com
Carol Queen, PhD, is staff sexologist at Good Vibrations
    education@goodvibes.com
Chronic Sex aims to open up discussion about how illness

and disability affect peoples' lives, specifically focusing on self-love, self-care, relationships, sexuality, and sex itself –
www.chronicsex.org

Dara Hoffman-Fox is a world-renowned gender therapist who helps people all across the gender and sexuality spectrum get in touch with themselves. Dara is also non-binary, so knows both sides –
http://darahoffmanfox.com/

GLMA is an association of health providers focused on providing the best environments for LGBTQ+ patients and providers - www.glma.org/

Hedonish is a site run by Rachael Rose, a sexuality educator who lives with a variety of health conditions including MCAS and vulvar pain –
http://hedonish.com/

Intimate Health Consulting provides teaching and consulting services to medical professionals around sexuality, abuse survivors, and more –
www.intimatehealthconsulting.com/

JoEllen Notte is a sex educator who focuses on sex, mental health, and how none of us are broken –
www.redheadbedhead.com/

Kait Scalisi, MPH, is a sexuality educator living with Crohn's and Ankylosing Spondylitis –
www.passionbykait.com/

ORCHIDS, the Organization for Research on Chronic Illness, Disability, and Sexuality, focuses on how we can improve sexuality research through an intersectional and inclusive lens –
https://orchidsresearch.org/

Project Prepare trains medical students to provide

outstanding patient care around sexual health –
www.projectprepare.org/

Internet addresses are current at time of publication.

ACKNOWLEDGEMENTS

From Iris:
I would like to first thank Jenny Palter for coming to my lectures, interviewing me, and encouraging me to share this important subject with a larger audience. I would like to thank my girls Madelyn, Lilly, Gloria, Brittany, and Zorah, for living with a mom who studied and obsessed about sexual health for all of their childhoods. Their support was constant and loving. I would also like to thank Christopher, my husband, for being my soul mate and teaching me what real intimacy means.

From Jenny:
I want to express my heartfelt thanks to Iris, for giving me the opportunity to make this long-held dream a reality. It has been a fun and highly educational collaboration, to say the least! Appreciation also goes out to my readers, Chris Title, Teri Allbright Wildrick, Alex Cielo, and Dr. Robert Phillips, for all the suggestions and support. Nick Courtright and his colleagues at Atmosphere Press made the publishing process seem like a family project, for which I am so grateful. Finally, my never-ending thanks to Francisco Quintanilla, for always being there.

ABOUT ATMOSPHERE PRESS

Atmosphere Press is an independent, full-service publisher for excellent books in all genres and for all audiences. Learn more about what we do at atmospherepress.com.

We encourage you to check out some of Atmosphere's latest releases, which are available at Amazon.com and via order from your local bookstore:

Geometry of Fire, nonfiction by Paul Warmbier

Chasing the Dragon's Tail, nonfiction by Craig Fullerton

Pandemic Aftermath: How Coronavirus Changed Global Society, nonfiction by Trond Undheim

Great Spirit of Yosemite: The Story of Chief Tenaya, nonfiction by Paul Edmondson

My Cemetery Friends: A Garden of Encounters at Mount Saint Mary in Queens, New York, nonfiction and poetry by Vincent J. Tomeo

Change in 4D, nonfiction by Wendy Wickham

Disruption Games: How to Thrive on Serial Failure, nonfiction by Trond Undheim

Eyeless Mind, nonfiction by Stephanie Duesing

ABOUT THE AUTHORS

Iris Zink, BSN, MSN, ANP, RN-BC, has been a rheumatology Nurse Practitioner for 18 years. She is the immediate past president of the Rheumatology Nurses Society, where she was president from 2015 to 2017. She has traveled extensively lecturing on a variety of topics pertaining 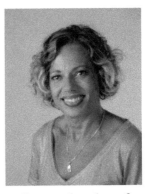 to arthritis, women and autoimmune disease, laughter for healing, and intimacy and chronic disease. Ms. Zink has published many times on topics about patient care and intimacy. She co-authored the chapters on HIV and arthritis, Osteoarthritis, and Ehlers Danlos Hypermobility syndrome in *Core Curriculum for Rheumatology Nursing.* She also co-authored, with Ms. Palter, the chapter on Sexual Health in *Chronic Rheumatic Diseases* in the forthcoming edition. Ms. Zink is adjunct faculty at Michigan State University and Grand Valley State University and a passionate teacher, lecturer, and caregiver. In 2016, she opened the first Nurse Practitioner-run early arthritis clinic in Michigan to provide access to care for those individuals who are under insured or uninsured. In 2017, she was honored to receive the Lupus Foundation of America's Inspirational Award for coining "PJ Day," which occurs every May 2 to raise money for research, education, and awareness of lupus. Iris's husband, Christopher Title, RRT, BSN, FNP is the co-founder of the clinic. He has been a nurse since 2002 and a Nurse Practitioner since 2015.

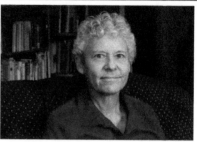

Jenny Thorn Palter, BS, is a writer and editor living in Western Maryland. From 1998 to 2018, she created educational materials and served as *Lupus Now* magazine editor at the Lupus Foundation of America. She previously collaborated with Ms. Zink on the "Sexual Health in Chronic Rheumatic Diseases" chapter for the Second Edition of the *Core Curriculum for Rheumatology Nursing*. Ms. Palter was diagnosed with Systemic Lupus in 1993, at age 35, after experiencing symptoms since adolescence, and with Fibromyalgia in 2015. Ms. Palter received her BS in journalism from Texas A&M University.

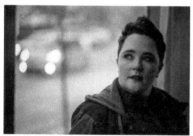

Kirsten Schultz, MS, is a rheumatology patient turned sex educator and a lifelong health nerd who has worked in the public health arena with a focus on chronic illnesses and disability. Kirsten has presented talks across North America in addition to working with patient organizations, pharmaceutical companies, and universities. Kirsten holds an MS in healthcare administration and runs research on patient engagement, sexuality, and healthcare. You can learn more about them and their work at kirstenschultz.org.

R. Mimi Secor, DNP, FNP-BC, FAANP, FAAN, has worked for 43 years as a Family Nurse Practitioner specializing in Women's Health. In addition to the credentials of Fellow in both the American Association of Nurse Practitioners (AANP) and the prestigious American Academy of Nursing (AAN), she earned her 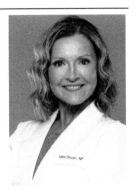 Doctorate in Nursing Practice (DNP) from Rocky Mountain University of Health Professions in Provo, Utah, in 2015. She is perhaps best-known as part of a dynamic mother-daughter duo, Dr. Mimi and Coach Kat, dedicated to helping women transform their lives by improving their health and fitness. Her international best-selling book that tells of her improbable journey is titled *Debut a New You: Transforming Your Life at Any Age* (Epic Author Publishing; 2017). Dr. Mimi resides in Onset, Massachusetts.

Photo of Iris and Chris on page 112 taken by Terri Shaver

Printed in the USA
CPSIA information can be obtained
at www.ICGtesting.com
LVHW060512201123
764349LV00023B/1502